DRAWN TOGETHER

Maintaining Connections and Navigating Life's Challenges with Art

A Father Daughter Story

Roar & Katarina Thorsen

ROAR'S DEDICATION

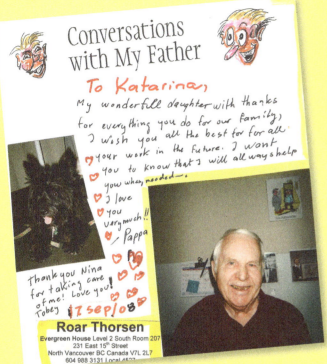

This book is dedicated to my daughter, Katarina.

"Katarina, you are not only my daughter, but also my best friend and my inspiration. It's amazing to have a daughter like you. I cannot even count the number of times you have helped me with doctors, hospital visits, etc. You have always been beside me. You have acted as my advisor. You have always been my guide, especially when I've been discussing difficult situations with you.

I've been in residential care for five years and very often you have asked, "Are you OK?" My answer: "I've never had it so good." Working with you is a blessing. In talking with you, I get the feeling that nothing is impossible.

Another wonderful thing is that you helped me rediscover my art. We always sit together and discuss each picture. You never criticize my work. When each new day comes, I feel good, since I know that you will take care of everything, continuing in the same style.
Do not be sentimental.
LIFE IS LIFE. LET'S GO."

Pappa

KATARINA'S DEDICATION

For my children Anna and Julian and my nephew, Henrik- the next generation.
For my father's caregivers, whose selfless work does not go unnoticed.
For Julie and Greg Salisbury, my collaborators at Influence Publishing, for making dreams come true.

ACKNOWLEDGMENTS

I would like to acknowledge the wonderful support we have received from so many people who have enriched our lives beyond words. Without you, this project would not have reached fruition. – Katarina Thorsen

Thank you's to:

Karin Thorsen, my mother- who led by example and taught me how to be a caregiver and to love unconditionally. I miss you, Mom. The next one is for you.

Tobey, my dog, my "life partner" and Dad's therapy. His presence has been essential.

My family: Anders Thorsen, Charmaine Crooks, Fredrik Thorsen, Cher Hanusiak, Henrik Thorsen, Anna Thorsen and Julian Bowers, for their constant love and support. Thank you, Cher, for your profound conversations and Fredrik for teaching me the power of the story and making time and room for me to work, and for collaborating on this book.

Julian, my son, whose documentary, *Drawn Together*, perfectly and masterfully captures the spirit of his grandfather. Julian's support throughout my personal journey is nothing less than life saving.

J. Lastoria and Julian for creating extraordinary original music for the documentary.

The care-aides, housekeepers, nurses, doctors and technicians at Evergreen House Residential Care Centre and Lions Gate Hospital for outstanding care and service.

Dr. Carolyn Gilbert, for her extraordinary attention, care and advocacy.

Kimberly Borgfjord, whose humor, grace and sensitivity when caring for my father, stands out as a shining example for her profession.

Jacquie Man, "China Tiger," whose boisterous humour has kept Dad's spirits soaring!

Eduardo Bursalona, housekeeper, who would check in with Dad and I regularly and chat as we worked away on our book at our special table in the northwest corner of the cafeteria. His visits meant so much to us.
The housekeeping gang at their 5 pm and 7 pm breaks in the cafeteria whose love for Dad and sense of humor fills my heart with joy. They would regularly yell "Lucky Guy!" to Dad and he would growl and shake his fist back at them in camaraderie.

The baristas at the cafeteria, for making the best hot black coffee. We drank copious amounts.

Lucca Hallex, for the title of the book and for her intuitive wisdom.

InspireABook® Mastermind participants: Hannelore, Dr. Nelie Johnson, Lucca Hallex, Sharon Watts, Nathalie Dignard, Carolle MacIntosh, Leslie Fierling and Brad MacIntosh, whose feedback shaped the book.

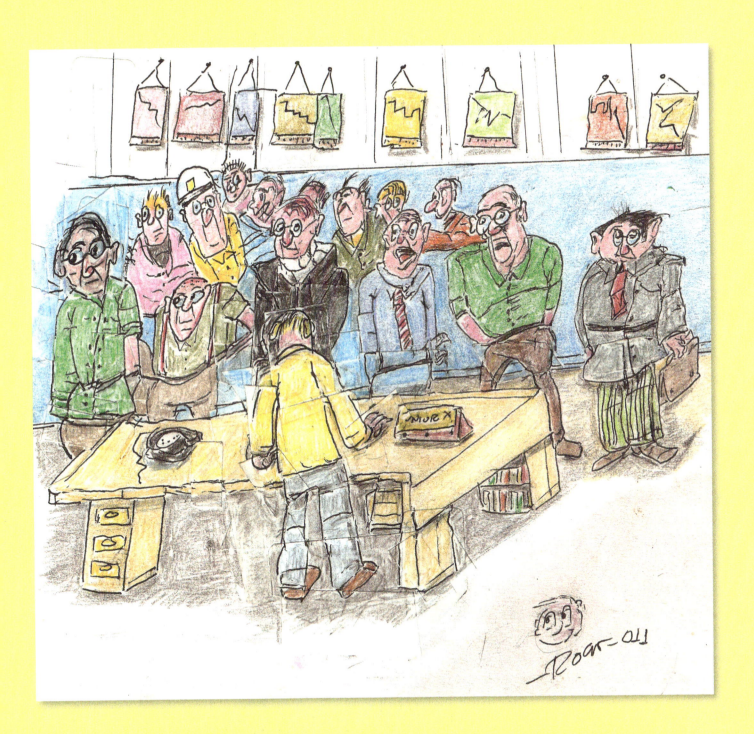

Our Indiegogo funders who helped bring the book to its final stage: Lynn Gosnell, Anna Coffin, Loretta Cella, Douglas Bruce Clement, Anders Thorsen, Ian Powell, Ashleigh Medlam, Anonymous #1, John Baechler, Margareta and Magnus Ericson, Peter Ericson, Evelyn Wong, Gretchen Miller, Matthew Krinbring, Julie Salisbury, Jay Couvillon, Norman Berglund, Darcy Guenette, Deb Sreejita, Joseph Killian, Annika Orwald Printz, Robert Nadeau, Hannah, Anonymous #2, Oliver McTavish-Wisden, Glen Winter, Matthew Roy, Paula Cook, Laura Mack, Mark Adams, Anna Thorsen, Cher Hanusiak, Desmond Reid, Josh Langston, Fredrik Thorsen, Anne Banner, Robyn and Joal Wishart, Caren Hall, Krongtong Boonprakong and Justine Tan.

Our supporters on Facebook and Twitter who helped spread the word.

The Heart and Stroke Foundation for providing invaluable information and support after my father's stroke.
.
Cheryl Bain, an expert on recreational therapy for seniors and whose talents and spirit inspires me every day. We were dancers when we met and became fast friends. She remains my dearest friend to date.

Laura Mack, my friend and mentor, whose ability to connect and netweave people together has led to amazing opportunities for me. She can make anyone feel better by just the turn of a phrase. I treasure her.

Gretchen Miller, my art therapy mentor and hero.

Darcy Guenette, who fed me, sewed sock monkeys with me, journal-ed with me, confided in me, listened to me, encouraged me and got me through days when I thought I couldn't take another step.

Jay Fisher, for encouraging me to own it.

Julie Salisbury of Influence Publishing. This book would not be possible without her.

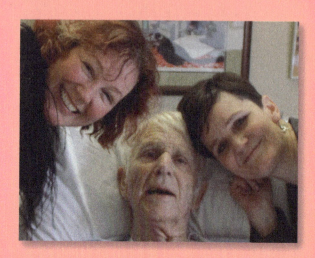

TABLE OF CONTENTS

There is no beginning. I've tried to invent one but it was a lie and I don't want to be a liar. This story will end where it began, in the middle. A triangle or a circle. A closed loop with three points.
Janna Levin

It becomes a journey of insight, of symbolic stages.
Oliver Sacks

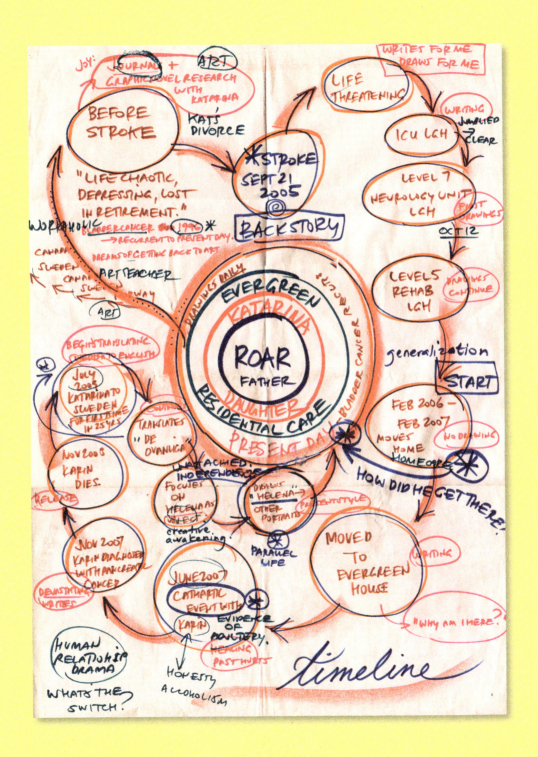

FOREWORD

Art washes from the Soul the dust of everyday life.
Pablo Picasso

Drawn Together is a love story written between father and daughter reflecting on the healing power of art therapy and human relationship. It has affirmed the therapeutic gift of art through creative process and self-discovery. In my role as a recreation therapist, I have observed Katarina in action sharing art therapy techniques with older adults challenged with dementia and Alzheimer's. Their artistic experiences awakened their creativity, cognition, sense of purpose, social connections and spirituality– the list goes on.

Katarina and her father, Roar, show us that the process of art can influence all aspects of a person's life. The creative process is, instinctively, part of who we all are. *Drawn Together* inspires possibilities of removing barriers due to disabilities and illness, inviting us to heal and grow through artistic exploration and creative freedom. It is a legacy of love.

Cheryl Bain
Recreation Therapist
Vancouver, BC

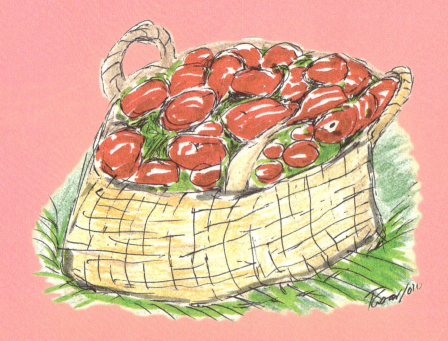

HOW TO USE THIS BOOK

READ IT. SHARE IT. BE INSPIRED.

Who is this book for?

DRAWN TOGETHER is for anyone who craves to awaken to their own gifts and who desire to connect with others in new and profound ways that are mutually beneficial and stimulating.

Why do I need it?

DRAWN TOGETHER is a call to action to collect stories and to create a legacy. Don't wait for the ultimate moment, for that moment is here NOW and it is fleeting.

What will this book teach me?

DRAWN TOGETHER inspires readers to awaken to their own gifts and to facilitate artistic expression in others. It illustrates that a life-threatening event can be a means to finding a richer life and that art can, indeed, heal.

How does the book work?

We learn by example, and DRAWN TOGETHER teaches that creativity can enrich relationships. This book is one father-daughter story, but it encourages, through text and image, all of us to build deeper connections.

INTRODUCTION

While we have the gift of life, it seems to me the only tragedy is to allow part of us to die whether it is our spirit, our creativity, or our glorious uniqueness.

Gilda Radner

Katarina's journal entry:

I walked up the stairs to check on my father. I couldn't hear the TV, so I assumed he might be asleep or reading the paper. I found him sitting at his desk, just staring straight ahead. Just staring. His papers untouched. His coffee cold. His TV off. His shoulders deflated. He had stopped. Simply stopped. It was time to make a drastic change. His needs were beyond what we could provide him at home. I went against his wishes and moved him to residential care, and I bought him a new set of pencils. That was February 2007. The other day my father told me he loves his life. "Why, Pappa? What changed?" "It was a pencil. It was you. It is us."

My father has the most appropriate name: Roar. I seldom call him *Dad*. I call him *Pappa*. For our purposes here, I refer to him as *Roar*.

Roar suffered a massive stroke in 2005 that left him paralyzed on the left side. His recovery was difficult and awe-inspiring. His tenacity, stubbornness, strength, creativity, his one good arm and most importantly, his humour allowed him to eventually forge a life within a residential care facility that became both fulfilling and rewarding.

It is his art that has provided Roar with a much-needed connection to the world. I do take some credit in facilitating this connection, pulling Dad out of what Proust referred to as "the abyss of unbeing." This was such a natural thing to do as all my life my father has nurtured my creative spirit and we have kept our connection rich through journaling, drawing and mutual encouragement. This connection has allowed us to support each other through a variety of life challenges. Despite his health concerns, my father wakes each day now excited about his next drawing or our next typing session. Ours is a deep father-daughter connection and, I dare say, it may be a very unique connection. I love that old man!

In the spirit of simplicity and authenticity, I have decided on a personal approach to presenting his work and our

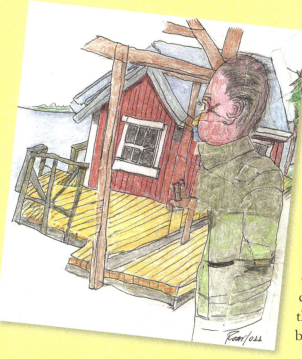

journey. My father has a distinct way of expressing himself and my intent is to allow his unique voice to come through in these pages. Since starting this project in 2009, we have accumulated a large collection of Roar's "post-stroke drawings." They are magical sketches exuding child-like honesty and reflecting masterful mark making. They charm and inspire the viewer and deserve to be shared with the world.

I have collected our journal entries and chosen specific drawings by Roar that best illustrate the theme in each chapter. I have purposely not dated the journal entries, for they illustrate specific moments and reflections and the dates felt unimportant and distracting-except in Chapter 10, as my father faces the final chapter in his life and chronology felt important. The book follows the original mind map created for the book during a weekend writer's course with Julie Salisbury of Influence Publishing. My father loves this mind map so much; we decided to let it guide the shape of the book.

The book is divided into four main parts: Part One: Before the Stroke, Part Two: The Stroke, Part Three: Residential Care and lastly, a gallery of Roar's drawings and words of wisdom. Each chapter generally contains snippets of journal entries, drawings and assorted photos. Though the majority of the illustrations in the book are Roar's post-stroke drawings, Chapter Two contains samples of his early work. These make an interesting comparison as to how his mark making changed after September 21, 2005.

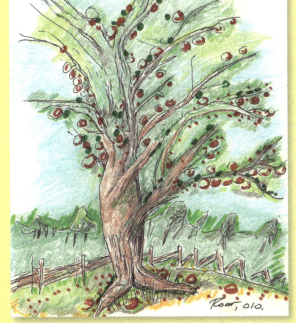

I've been wondering about the word *legacy* in regards to this book. Is it the need to *leave a legacy* that drives the work we do as artists? Is the drive to leave a mark simply our personal strive for immortality? If our legacy is this little book, inspiring only one person who comes across it, then my father and I agree our work is done.

At this writing, my father is facing a new chapter in his life as he battles metastatic bladder cancer. His spirit remains vigorous and tenacious despite his pain and we are energized as we plan our next project. For that is how we stay connected and alive. Work. Art. Love.

I want to be old since I think it is interesting to live.
Roar Thorsen

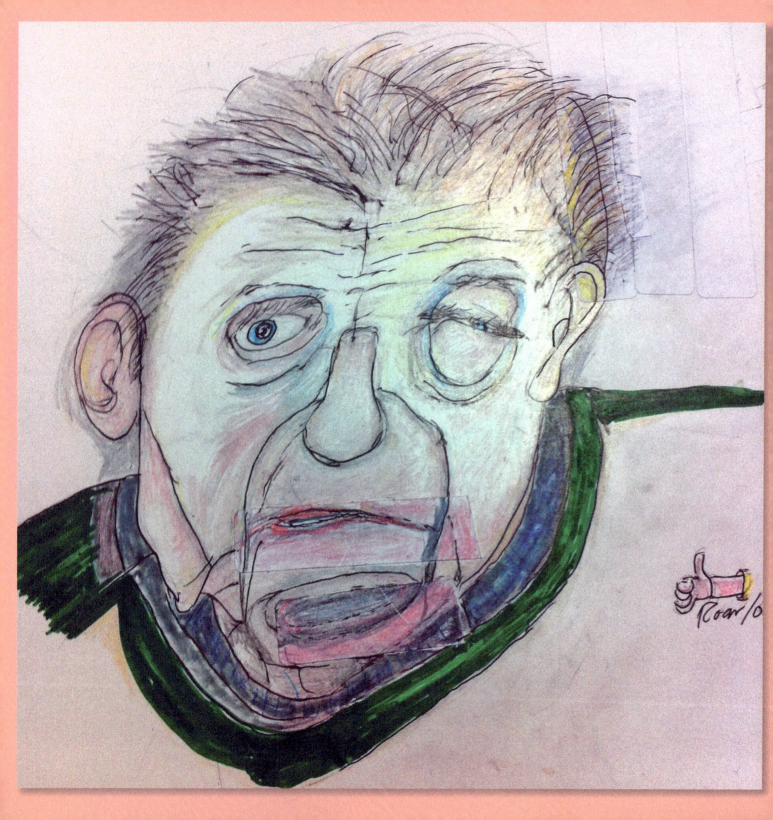

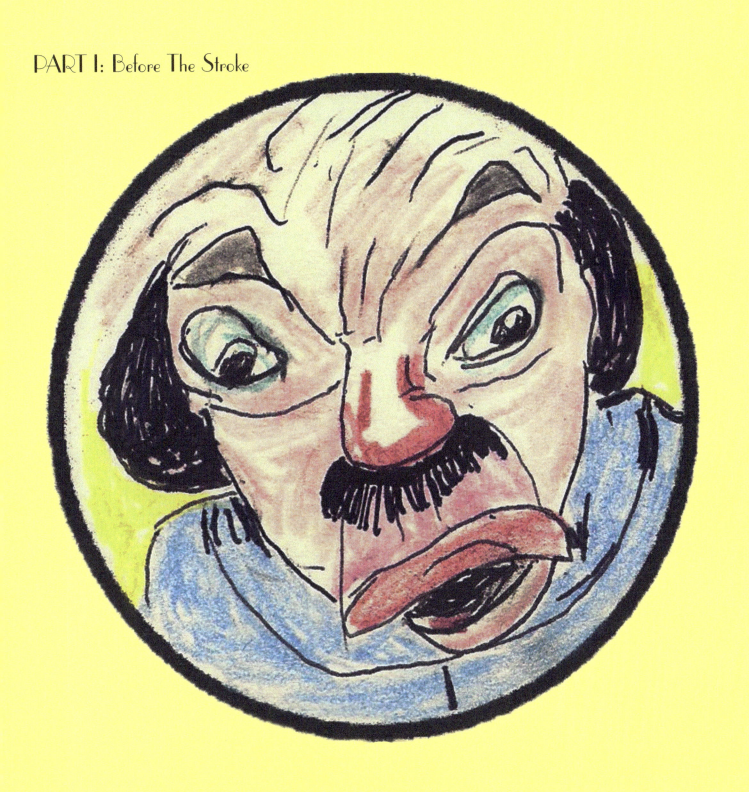

CHAPTER ONE: Present Day

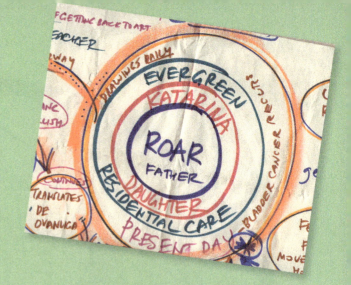

We must be willing to let go of the life we planned
so as to have the life that is waiting for us.
Joseph Campbell

Roar's journal entry:

One day in September 2005, I suddenly found myself in the world of strokes, with loss of strength in my left arm and leg. After a difficult recovery, I told myself, I do not have time for this nonsense. Since my brain was still working, I decided immediately to get back to my normal life and continue my usual artwork. I was often asked how I could recover so quickly after such an experience? I just think, so what? What's the big deal?

Three weeks after the stroke, I was already drawing as part of my recovery process. A year and a half after my stroke, I decided, in discussion with my family, to enter a residential care center. Here, I rediscovered my love of drawing. I told myself: I do not want to just sit around wasting time! I refused to become one of those old and sick people. In my new life, I have little time to chat as I concentrate on being creative and inspirational!

What keeps me going is the encouragement from my family, especially my daughter Katarina, since we both love art. Through the work and support of Katarina, I have been working on several volumes of illustrated text, and I could not be more inspired. In short, art has put me back in the race.

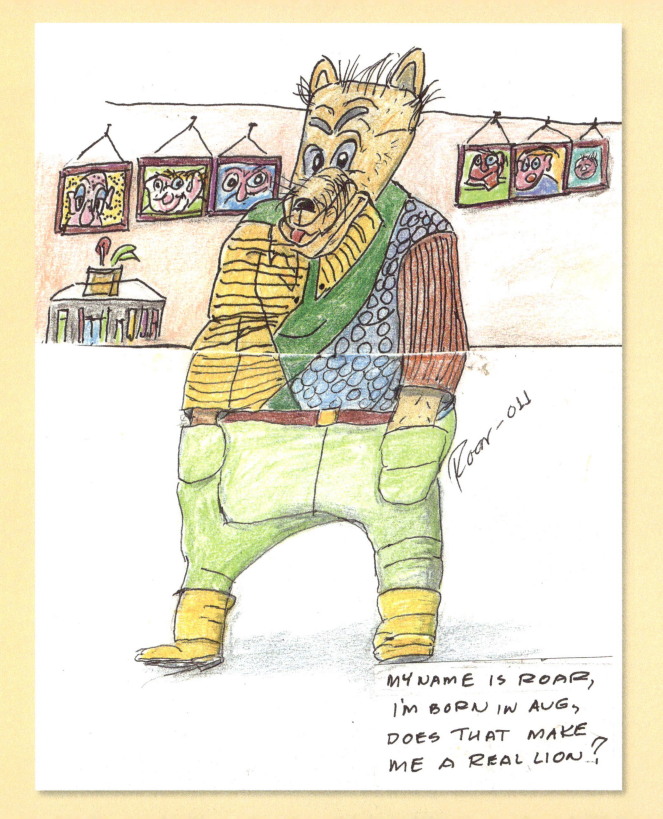

Katarina's journal entry:

How do you start a book? Where do you start? Start where you are. And right now I am sitting in a chair beside my father's bed. He's eating ribs from White Spot and I'm about to give him his strawberry ice cream. His back has a bad spasm. He's not allowed to drink his whiskey due to the muscle relaxant. But he's watching the news and eating his ribs and sipping on his drink. I'm tucked in the corner writing in my journal. Tobey is asleep under the bed. His plate (Roar's rejected hospital dinner) is licked clean. My father's wheelchair is tucked into his desk. And his shoes sit under the TV table. His catheter hangs under the bed and I watch blood clots move slowly through the tube. I never thought I would hate the color russet brown. But I do now.

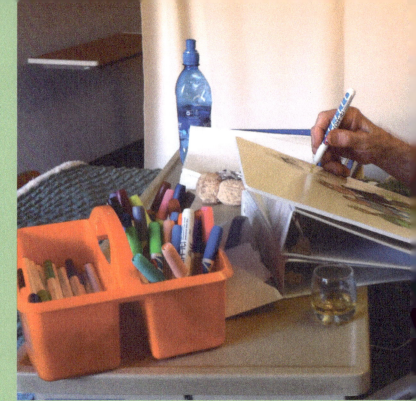

My father is chewing on a salt and peppered rib and enjoying a pain free moment. His desk has unread newspapers that he needs to sort through. His caregiver, Kim, moved the catheter tube from the right to the left to allow gravity to do its work. The latest drawing hangs on the wall along gallery row. My throat closes up a bit to quell a cry that threatens to burst the peaceful moment. The marks he makes on paper, the tenacity at which he stays with a drawing, illustrates the way Roar has lived his life. He just doesn't know what giving up means.

The fridge is humming and my father is now moving his feet, enjoying the release of pain from his medication and enjoying his strawberry ice cream. The barista at the hospital café is excited about this book and I promised her we'd have a launch party at our favorite table in the cafeteria. That table. It's an essential part of this book. It's where Roar and I have held our meetings for 5 years now, working together on our art, typing our notes, analyzing our lives, sharing our ups and downs, watching Swedish movies, drinking endless cups of coffee, dreaming of sharing Roar's drawings with the world.

Our little life together is simply about father and daughter connection, a deep love and respect for each other, avarice for the creative process, a mutual love of research, a common ground and understanding and just two people holding onto each other, riding the waves of life.

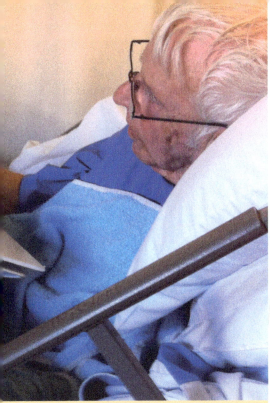

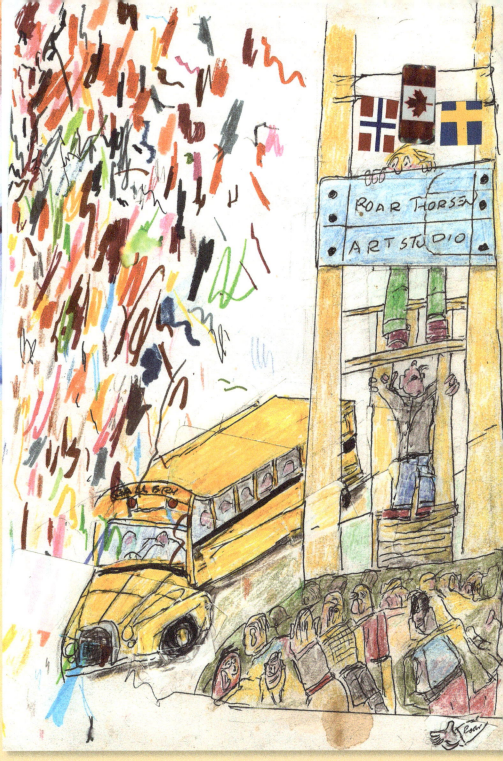

The roommate just fell in the bathroom, so I ran to the front desk and they are using the medilift to transfer him back to bed. Elizabeth is yelling *help me* over and over again, as usual, in the hallway and my father just yelled *shut up* to her! He's now changing channel on his TV and the evening is settling in. For what it is, it's good. Together a routine has been built and we thrive on that routine. We know what to expect from each other.

I know what Roar needs to keep his life puttering along, what needs to be in the drawer, what needs to be in the fridge and what needs to be on his desk. But it's art that keeps us both going- the routine of the unexpected and the joy of discovering something new. It's time to pack up and to say good night. My father seems cozy and more at ease. I admit that right now I am exhausted by grief and I know the only thing to get me through tonight is to go home and draw.

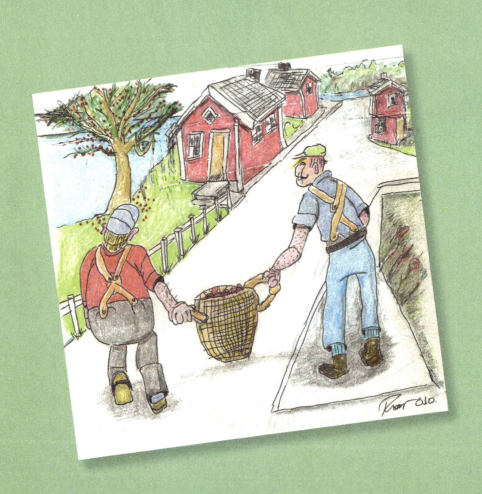

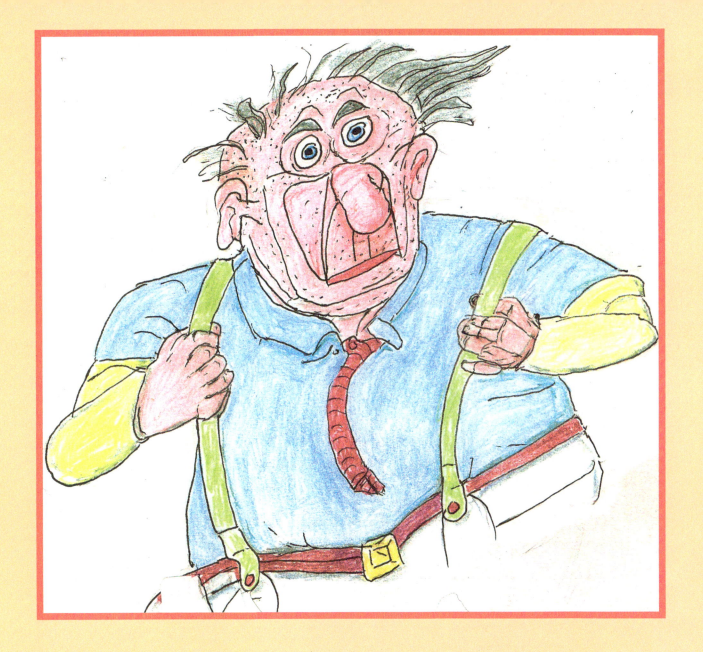

I am satisfied with my life, even if I'm not happy with everything.
Roar Thorsen

CHAPTER TWO: Roar's History

Through a tremulous prism, I distinguish the features of relatives and familiars, mute lips serenely moving in forgotten speech.
Vladimir Nabokov

Roar's journal entry:

I have drawn all my life.

As a small boy in Sarpsborg, Norway, many stories were read to me. As far as I remember, I entered Kindergarten at age 6. I started with pencil and paper from instruction and ideas by the teacher. She taught in a simple, natural way, with optimism and creativity, often by reading from books. By flicking through picture books, I got a better understanding of creating art. The books inspired me. The more I read and looked at the pictures, the more I tried to draw like that myself.

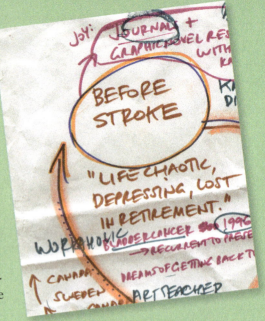

I remember one day, when I was about at 7, Mom and Dad told me that we were going to the cinema to see Disney's *Three Little Pigs*. In the beginning, I was scared since I was sitting in the aisle seat and I had been told that the film would show moving pigs. I asked if the pigs were going to come running in the aisles! They shut the lights off and we saw all the pigs running around on the screen. What the hell is this moving on the big screen? I was impressed. How do you do this? Little did I understand that by looking at these pigs on the movie screen, I would be inspired to draw cartoons. I started studying the drawings of Walt Disney.

By copying, suddenly I got into the Disney style of making characters, with their noses etc. In fact, in school, I always made Disney style drawings.

I showed a couple of drawings to the teacher that I had made at home. "Did you do this?" She asked for more. "I like the style you have chosen."

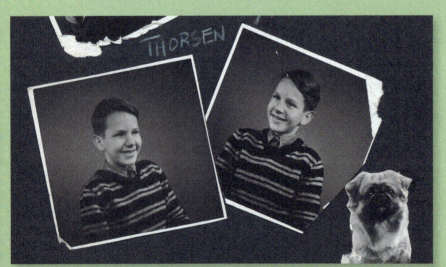

I finally built up the courage to send a letter to the Walt Disney Corporation telling him about my interest in his movies and books. To my astonishment a couple of weeks or months later, I got an envelope in the mail from Disney headquarters in Los Angeles. It contained a letter and two original drawings by Walt Disney's artists. They have unfortunately been lost over the years.

The walls in my room were covered with magazine cutouts and drawings. In the middle of these were those two Disney drawings.

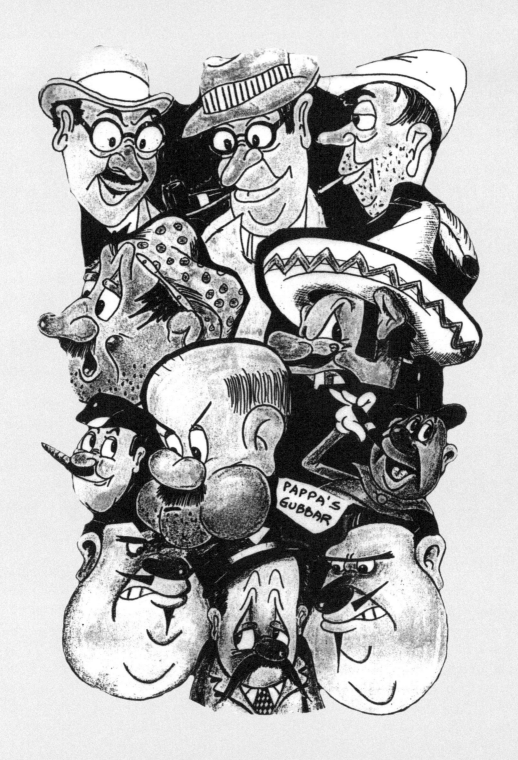

My dad's brother in Norway, Leif Hvål, was relatively famous. He was known for his ink drawings. His work contained different types of materials such as canvas, plywood and, of course, thick paper.

I often sat beside him, watching as he worked. When I visited exhibitions with my uncle, he explained the technical part of art. I learned a lot from him and he influenced my style at the time.

At 18, I found out that I had flunked Grade 12. They told me I had to repeat the grade. When I got home (we lived next door), Dad was waiting to hear how I did. I told him. He put me in the car and drove me to Skien and I had to work with my Grandpa and Grandma (on my mother's side). They had a general store with a little stone staircase and the house was painted yellow. The little store was in the middle of the town and the road was cobblestone. I was not allowed to be home in Sarpsborg. I was in Skien for a year. I helped my *Morfar* in the store. He was very nice. He would wear a vest and check his watch, which hung off a chain. The store smelled so damn good. I'll never forget it. They baked bread in the store. I got so many friends in Skien.

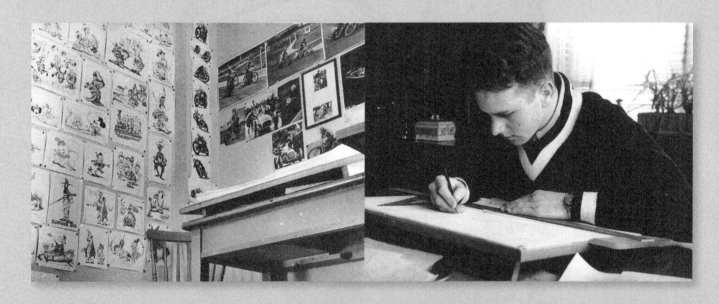

One block away from the store was a boat lock lifts in the Telemark Canal. After work I would head down there. All the local steamer traffic would go through the locks heading north with tourists. I would sit and watch. I became friends with the boss on the locks. The boat would unload tourists with all their luggage. The steamers would have long pipes. I spent most my time at the locks. The canal connected Notodden up North. That's where my uncle, Leif Hvål, lived.

I came back home after one year and I got called in to start Grade 12 again. That year went very well. I was best in the class and received highest marks. I was a veteran!

After graduating high school, one of my best friends suggested I look into the technical institute in Göteborg. I jumped right into what I wanted to do. Dad's connections also arranged a job at Volvo for a few months in

Göteborg (in the engineering department). Few weeks later I was fed up with the mass production. There was no individualism or encouragement. I traveled through Europe with my best friend around this time.

After 3 years abroad, I returned home. Dad searched out jobs for me. Dad's friend introduced me to his friends in the forest industry. I started in one of Norway's biggest papermills in Sarpsborg. I became very good friends with all the drafters. We drew by hand with a pencil!

After about 6 months, one of my friends moved to Sweden. He left the engineering office. A few weeks after he left, he called and told me to get my butt over to Sweden as there were plenty of jobs. The whole family cried. *Our son is leaving the country!* That was my first real step towards my independence and adventure.

Article in a forest industry newsletter circa 1970:

Roar Thorsen was born in Sarpsborg, Norway, August 8, 1930. After completing his education, he started work in the workshop at Borregaard, the largest pulp and paper mill in Norway. Then he did project design work for pulp and paper machines.

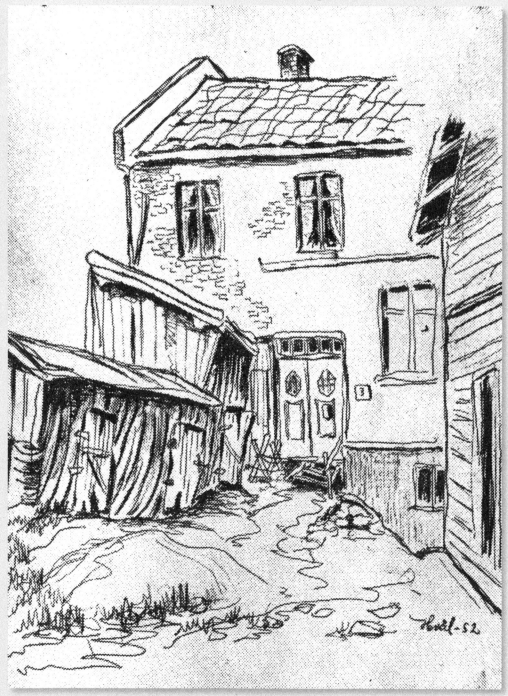

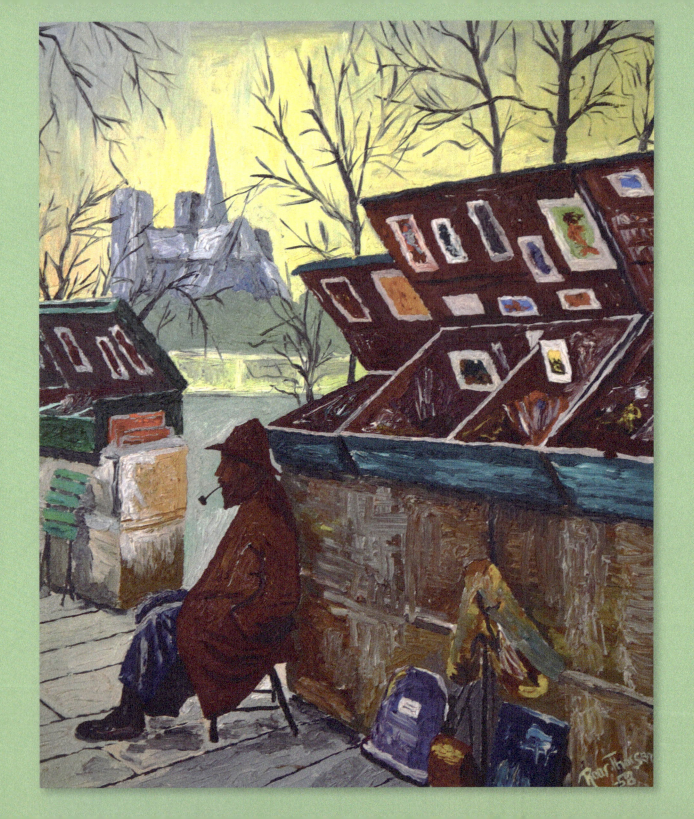

In 1949, he took two years out for military service with the Allied Forces in Germany. Roar moved to Sweden in 1955 where he met Karin, the future Mrs. Thorsen. For five years Roar worked as a project designer and engineer at Skoghallsverken and mill of the Uddeholm Company. He then moved on to the Billerud Company, 20 miles away as a project engineer at their paper mills. When Billerud started a sawmill expansion program in 1963, Roar was appointed a project engineer. "My first assignment was the Hällefors mill," says Roar. "It was completely rebuilt in nine months. The second job was at the Gruvön mill, which now has an annual production of 90 million board feet. That took a year to complete. I might add that Hällefors and Gruvön are now called Sweden's American mills.

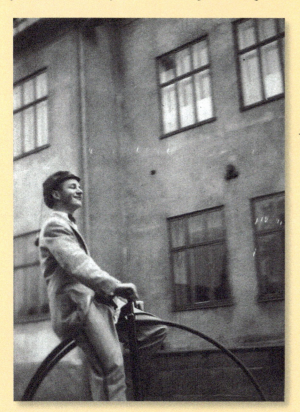

Not long after the Gruvön mill was completed the President of the Bulkey Valley Company, Derek Currie, visited Billerud. Roar was his guide for the two sawmills. Thorsen didn't realize it at the time, but from then on he was a marked man.

As Project Engineer for the Houston lumber mill, Roar Thorsen has the big job of equipping it with the most efficient sawmilling machinery and controls available. Then he has to make sure they all work well together.

About Christmas time the Thorsens will be moving up to Houston, British

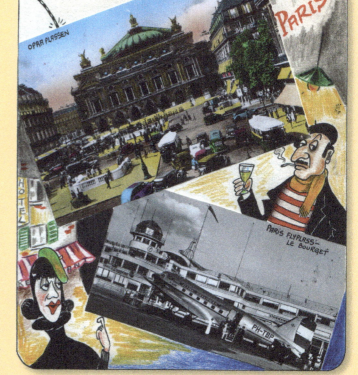

Columbia, Canada where they have bought a lot in Mountain View Park. They're looking forward to the move, because they think life in Houston will be very much like life in the mill towns in Sweden.

At the moment Roar and his family are living in a North Vancouver garden apartment. So far Roar hasn't had much chance to participate in one of his favorite sports, cross-country skiing. The whole family used to go cross-country skiing and little Fredrik used to ride in the pulka. A pulka is a kind of sled pulled along by a rope fastened to the shoulders. He also enjoys car-racing– as spectator sport– and fishing. Roar's main hobby is painting. "I do oils mostly, and some pen and ink drawings," he explained. "I also like drawing cartoons and had quite a lot of them published in the Billerud News."

   As a result of an exhibition in an art store, Roar sold several of his paintings. But although he finds his hobby fascinating and at times profitable, Roar Thorsen has no desire to earn his living by painting. "It's much safer to work as a Project Engineer for Bulkey Valley," he says, "and the income is steadier!"

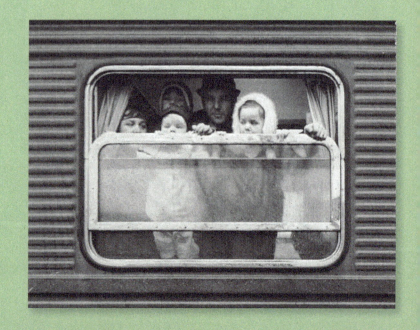

Roar's journal entry:

In 1975, I accepted another invitation to return to Sweden. Two years later we headed back to Canada. Each time I accepted a job offer, I always brought my family with me. I must say my family was very patient. In other words, no matter where we were, we always stayed together. All these moves have not harmed the children. In fact it made them smarter.

[Publication and author of article on Roar is unknown. Photocopy was found glued into one of Roar's journals.]

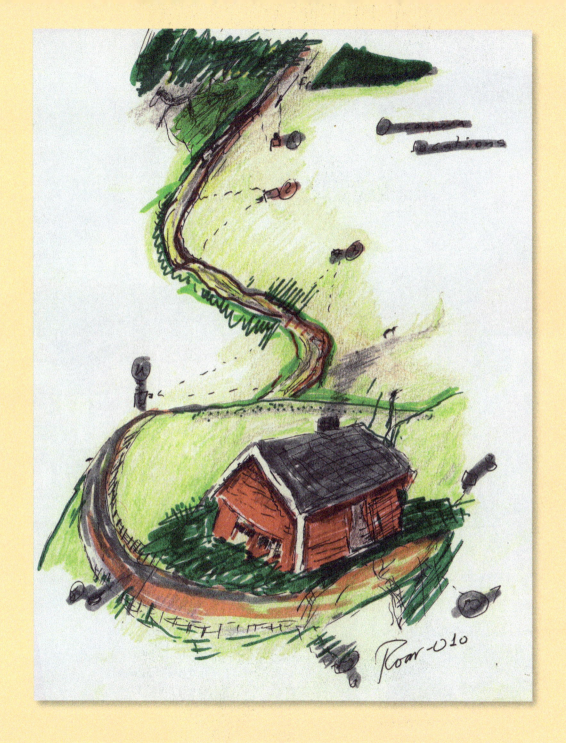

As I'm used to the view ever since childhood, I never noticed how beautiful it is.
Roar Thorsen

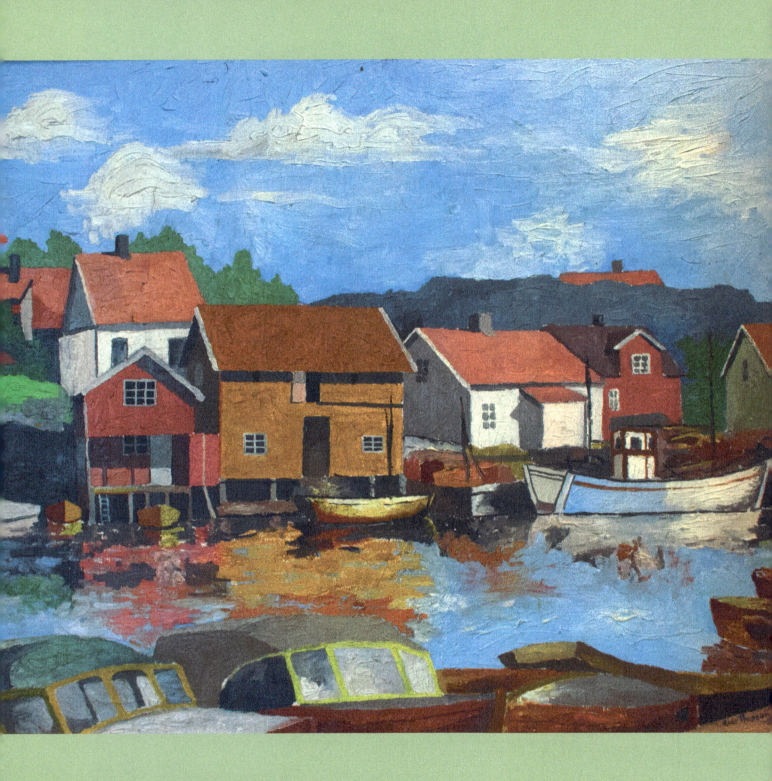

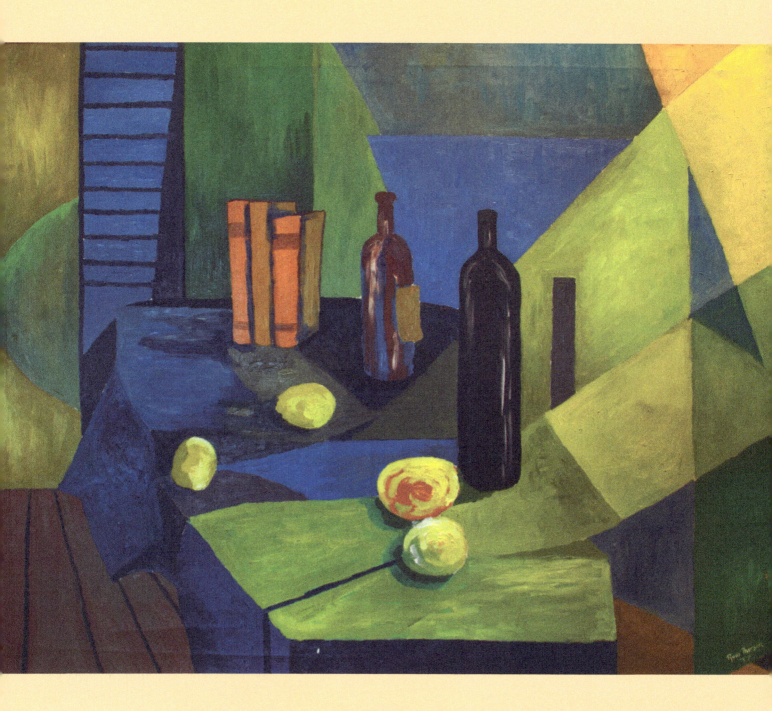

CHAPTER THREE: Father - Daugher Connection

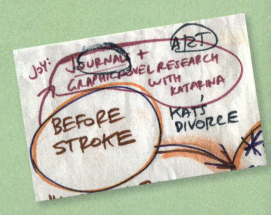

If we could see that everything, even tragedy, is a gift in disguise, we would then find the best way to nourish the soul
Elizabeth Kübler Ross

Katarina's journal entry:

I went to the storage room and pulled out some of the journals my father and I shared from 2002 to 2005. They are quite magical and they carried us through those tough years when I was struggling with the end of my marriage and Roar was struggling to find his identity while facing retirement and battling bladder cancer. There are more than a dozen collaborative journals and they are bursting at the seams.

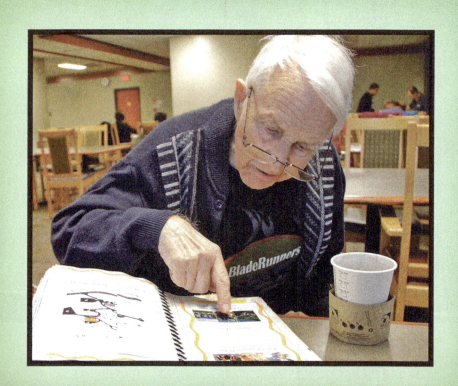

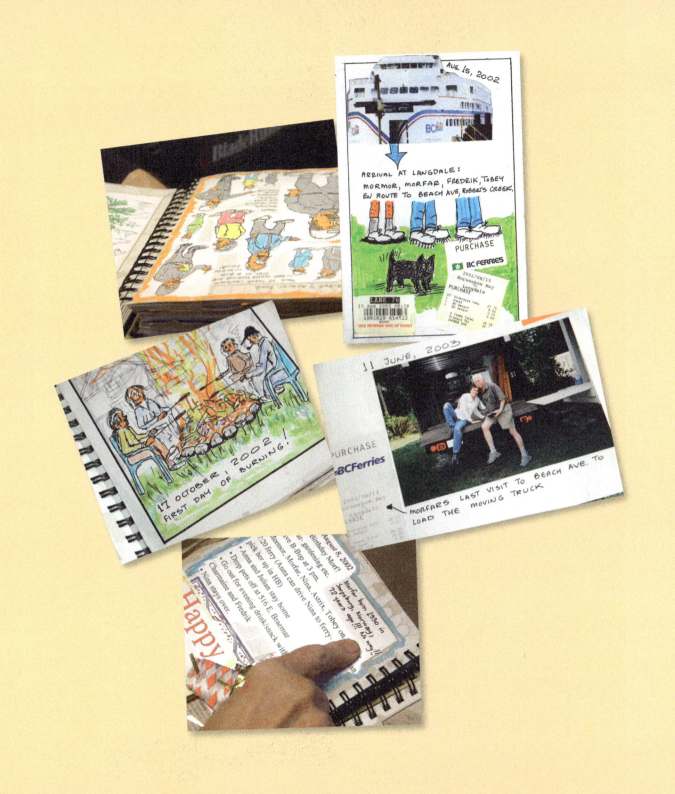

These were important lifelines for us. I was living on the Sunshine Coast and my parents were in North Vancouver. They would visit once a week and my father and I would alternate weeks writing and drawing in whatever the current journal was - Roar doing a few pages one week, and I would then take it and add to it. This kind of exchange carried on after Roar's stroke and we would also exchange news articles of interest.

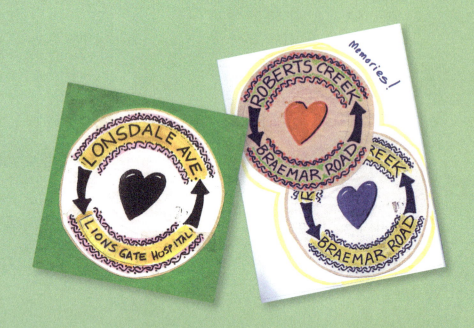

Our life together epitomizes the ultimate BIG-C word: Collaboration. Indeed, be it Crisis or Cancer or Chaos our father-daughter Connection remains all about

Creating-Commenting-Colluding-Contributing-Conversing-Communicating-Caregiving-Collecting and Coffee

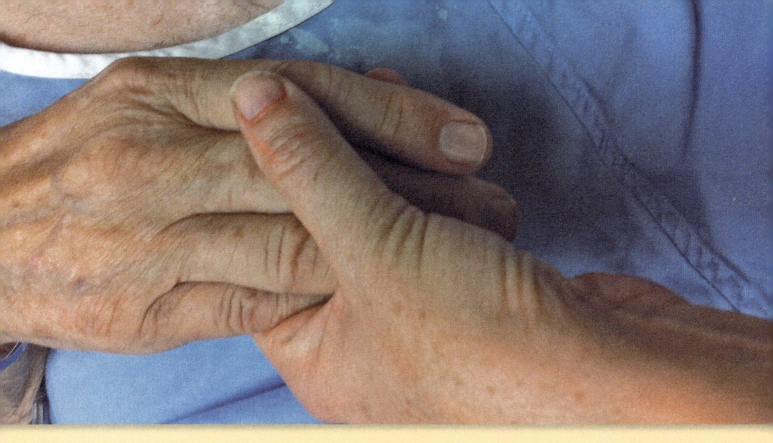

Roar's journal entry:

Advice to my daughter from a Viking Patriarch:

- Do not do too much yourself. You will burn out.
- Always delegate.
- Give proper instruction about what you need.
- Always remember- you are best.
- Always raise your voice in meetings. Being quiet shows that you are weak.
- Always be open to suggestions.
- Never take no for an answer.
- Always remember your own background.
- Always be a good listener to others.
- Always look for new positions and opportunities.
- Never look backwards, thinking that life was better before.

- Never forget the expression "I don't have time for this shit."
- You will always have Pappa for love, work, advice and encouragement etc.
- Always have an updated list of merits and accomplishments, containing everything from education to present.
- Include name and personal data: address, phone, email. Preferably a photo of yourself with a good background.
- Make a 5-year plan- where do you see yourself 5 years from now, 1 year from now, 1 month from now…?
- Never underestimate the power of the phrase, *please go fuck yourself.*
- Never forget that you are Daddy's girl.

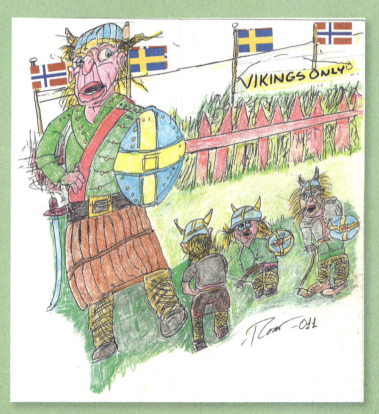

Katarina's journal entry:

After his stroke, I took in a new role with my father and found a way to fulfill both of us, and our artists within. Within those new limits, we recorded the process in our journals. We stay in the *now*, not getting trapped in a panic. There have been so many precious moments. There is so much left to do, or is there? We only have this moment right now. I am alive and so is my father.

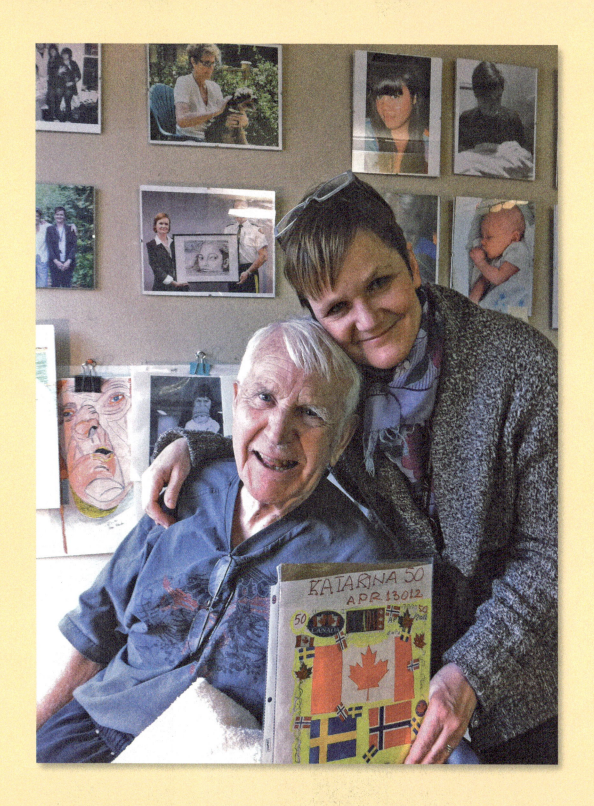

PART TWO: The Stroke

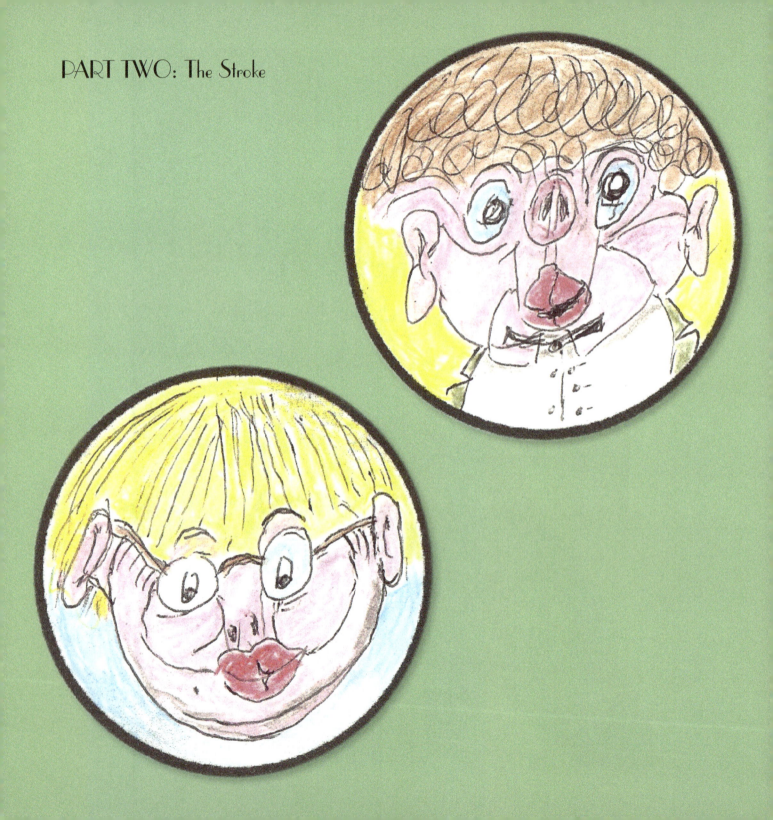

CHAPTER FOUR: September 21, 2005

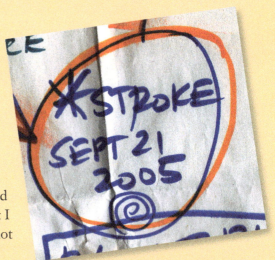

Change comes upon us, not slowly, gently evolving, within our control, but
suddenly, abruptly, within hours, sometimes moments, the course of our lives so
turned around, turned about, inside out
Fern Kupfer

Roar's journal entry:

When I got a stroke, it felt very strange, like I left my body and disappeared. I had needed to go to the doctor for a major checkup, but I never went. I was quickly taken to the hospital and they said, "He will not die. It's only part of the show."

Katarina's journal entry:

On September 21, 2005, we nearly lost Roar due to a severe bleeding stroke resulting in hemiplegia. Essentially, he was left paralyzed on his left side. He could not walk, but he could speak and his mind was clear. He became dependent on others for simple daily things such as transferring, toilet and dressing. Yut he has always been strong and stubborn, which has helped him immensely. The neurological unit was a messy hectic place. It made us feel vulnerable and desperate.

Within a few weeks of the stroke, I brought art supplies to my father's unit and his occupational therapist gave us a table to fit around his wheelchair.

His first drawing was most intriguing.

It clearly illustrates Roar's interpretation of his body. It is not a misrepresentation. It is an accurate depiction that Roar was not aware of his left side anymore.

I drew a simple sketch of a human body for him to copy to see if he could recognize the left side. The result was a charming drawing depicting his left side literally floating.

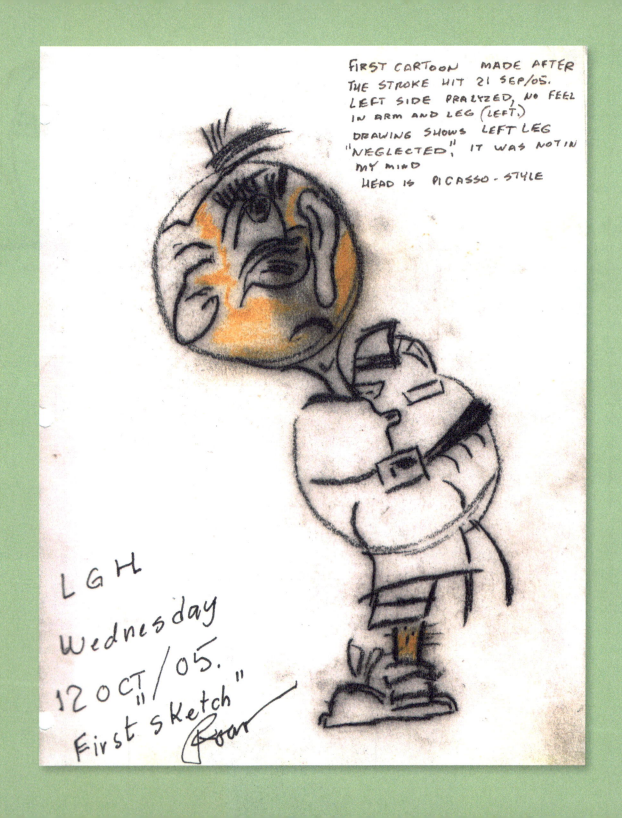

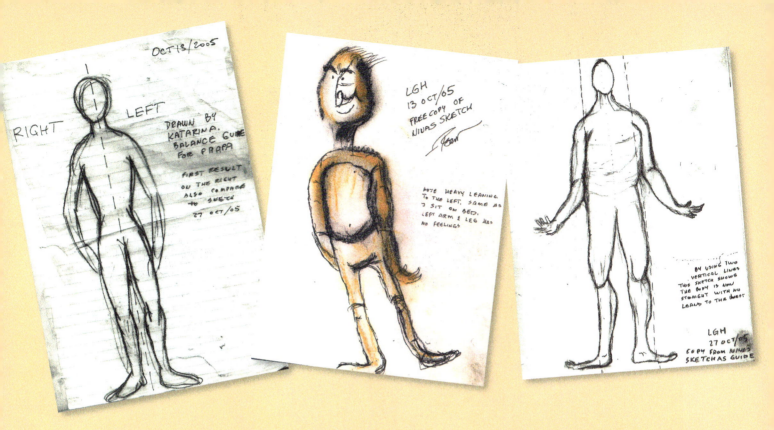

RIGHT LEFT

OCT 13/2005

DRAWN BY
KATARINA.
BALANCE GUIDE
FOR PRAPA

FIRST RESULT
ON THE RIGHT
ALSO COMPARE
TO SKETCH
27 OCT/05

LGH
13 OCT/05
FREE COPY OF
NINAS SKETCH

NOTE HEAVY LEANING
TO THE LEFT. SAME AS
I SIT ON BED.
LEFT ARM & LEG HAS
NO FEELINGS

BY USING TWO
VERTICAL LINES
THIS SKETCH SHOWS
THE BODY IS NOW
STRAIGHT WITH NO
LEANS TO THE LEFT

LGH
27 OCT/05
COPY FROM NINAS
SKETCH AS GUIDE

Two weeks later he did much better at recognizing the left side.

I recall that before my father's stroke I sensed a change was imminent. I had relocated to North Vancouver and my parents were living just a few blocks from me. My father and Tobey, the dog, would walk me home after my visits. We would say good night at Victoria Park. As my Dad turned back to walk home, I would stand and watch him. I did this for several months, sensing soon he would not be walking like that ever again.

On the day of the stroke, the family gathered at the hospital. We were there for most of the day. I know my mother spent the night in emergency. I recall coming back to her place to grab some things and the rest of the family were in the kitchen around the table. I was told they had voted me in charge. Oh, boy. It was time to start a new binder.

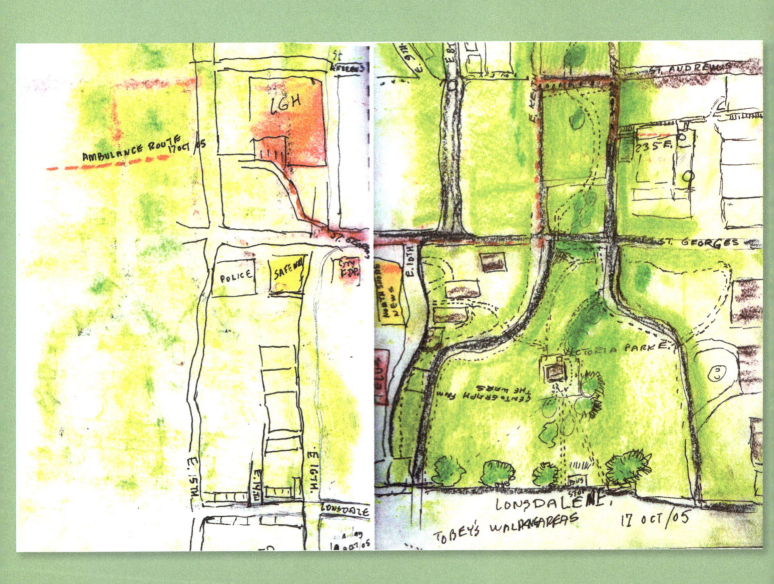

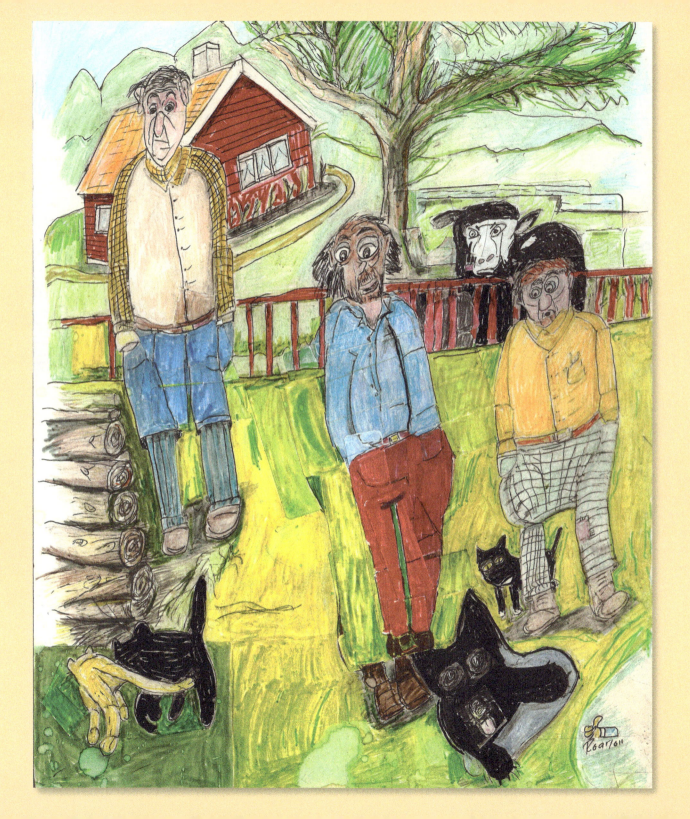

CHAPTER FIVE ICU: Neurology and Rehabilitation

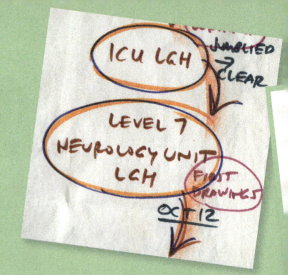

The normal frustrations of modern life are here multiplied and amplified.
E.B. White

Roar's journal entry:

What does recovery mean to me? Finding what you are looking for. Recovery means that you learn to live with it. You find out that it is no big deal, as long as you've got patience. Just keep on going.

I lost the feeling and ability to move my left arm, my left leg, the ability to walk, but I still have my brain. The handicap, which mainly affects the walking, doesn't affect the brain. So I was lucky.

I remember the first thing I said to my daughter- *let's get on with it. I've got no time to lie here.* My hobby really pushed me forward. No big deal. The only thing that changed is the left hand and leg. I'm physically disabled (for lack of a better word) and something in the body is no longer the same.

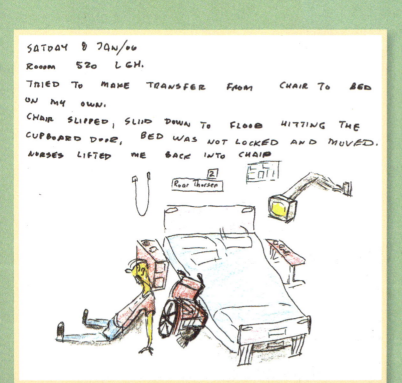

Many tell me I am really lucky and I agree. I can use my right hand as before. With that in mind, I do not lack in my enthusiasm to change something. That brings me right back to making drawings. I started to make drawings a few days after being released from the ICU..

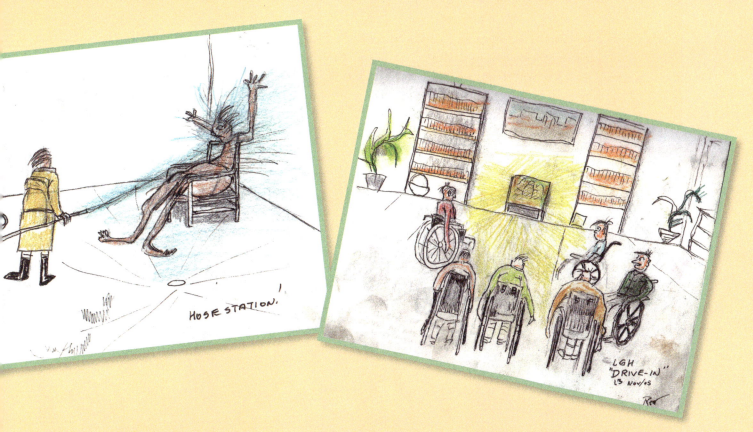

HOSE STATION!

LGH "DRIVE-IN" 13 NOV/05

Katarina's journal entry:

My father recorded daily life at the hospital in his drawings. He spent two weeks in neurological intensive care, then several weeks in the neurology ward. I found the place nightmarish. The fragility of the human skull and mind was evident everywhere. I believe that drawing allowed Roar both detachment and empowerment, making that foreign world, and his loss of independence, bearable.

After the neurology ward, my father was moved down two floors to the rehabilitation clinic.

On one hand, my father thrived there. He was given daily intensive physical therapy, relearned how to dress himself and made goals for the future. On the other hand, he was intensely lonely.

We visited often and I took him to the cafeteria and we worked on his drawings and exchanged our envelopes, yet my father's desire to go home was understandable.

In all honesty, the idea of fulfilling Roar's 24-7 physical needs overwhelmed the family. We knew it was impossible to provide him with the daily physical aide and therapy he required to maintain the gains he achieved in rehab.

I recorded my father's first visit home in 24 stills on a disposable camera. I wanted to ensure that he knew that we celebrated the moment. There were weekly visits home after that as we all adjusted. A few bumps along the road made us delay Roar's return home until February 2006.

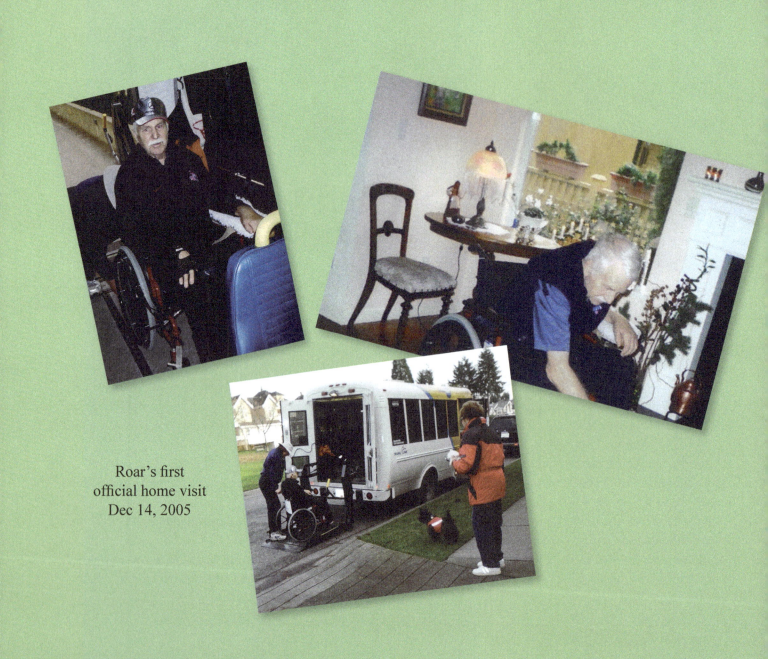

Roar's first
official home visit
Dec 14, 2005

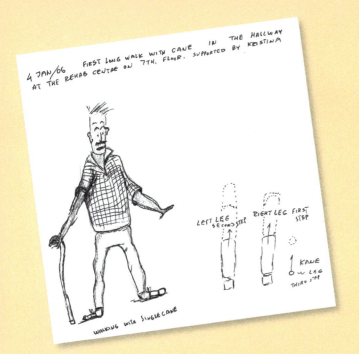

4 JAN/06 FIRST LONG WALK WITH CANE IN THE HALLWAY AT THE REHAB CENTRE ON 7TH. FLOOR. SUPPORTED BY KRISTINA

LEFT LEG SECOND STEP   RIGHT LEG FIRST STEP

CANE OW LEG THIRD STEP

WALKING WITH SINGLE CANE

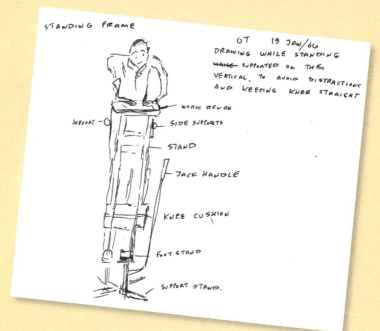

STANDING FRAME

OT 19 JAN/06
DRAWING WHILE STANDING WHILE SUPPORTED ON THE VERTICAL TO AVOID DISTRACTIONS AND KEEPING KNEE STRAIGHT

WORK BENCH
SUPPORT — SIDE SUPPORTS
STAND
JACK HANDLE
KNEE CUSHION
FOOT STAND
SUPPORT STAND.

Roar's journal entry:

Looking at photo album, I remember the Handydart itself. Same spot each time. I do not remember this event though, going back home for the first time after the stroke. I remember the garage at Keith Road. And the kitchen. I do remember that I cried. It was a natural reaction. I recall how confused I felt. All of a sudden I was home. I remember the living room. I remember the water cooler. And feeling confused. I remember the crawlspace. I don't recall that I still had a mustache!

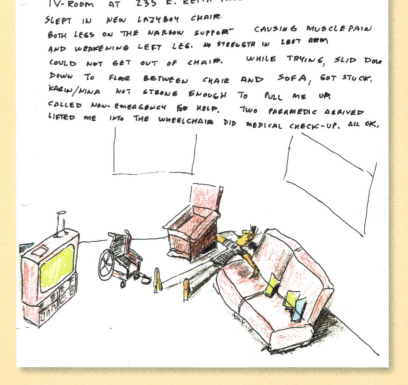

SUNDAY 9 JAN/06
TV-ROOM AT 235 E. KEITH HOUSE
SLEPT IN NEW LAZYBOY CHAIR.
BOTH LEGS ON THE NARROW SUPPORT CAUSING MUSCLE PAIN AND WEAKENING LEFT LEG. NO STRENGTH IN LEFT ARM COULD NOT GET OUT OF CHAIR. WHILE TRYING, SLID DOWN DOWN TO FLOOR BETWEEN CHAIR AND SOFA, GOT STUCK. KARIN/NINA NOT STRONG ENOUGH TO PULL ME UP. CALLED NON-EMERGENCY FOR HELP. TWO PARAMEDIC ARRIVED LIFTED ME INTO THE WHEELCHAIR DID MEDICAL CHECK-UP. ALL OK.

CHAPTER SIX: Moving Home

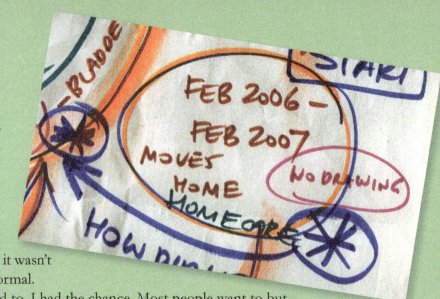

... And as this happened, I saw him retreat into solitude.
Michael Dorris

Roar's journal entry:

After the stroke, my goal became to get back to normal. That meant to go home. But it wasn't normal. It couldn't be. We had to reinvent normal.

I thought it was good to go home. I wanted to. I had the chance. Most people want to but they don't realize it's not the same. Despite the stair lifts, grab bars, super poles, wheelchairs and home care, I found out that home was no longer the same. In fact, I had a different feeling. This new life was not like I thought it would be. Everyone wants to go home, of course. That is typical. Although the house was nice, and my wife and family did their best, it just didn't work. My physical needs were overwhelming, so the atmosphere became stressful and this triggered a depression.

I had lived at Keith Road for only one year before the stroke. We had just downsized from our large family house to a townhouse. I then spent five months in the hospital. I didn't know I would only live at home for one year before moving to Evergreen House.

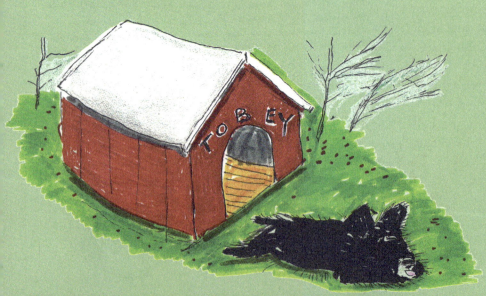

Initially, I was very happy to feel that I was coming home. It took time to adjust and be back with the family. But sitting around our dining table, I felt that this was different. One of my biggest goals was to adjust to a different environment. Although we were all together, I still had a feeling that I was not there yet. I slowly tried to garden again like before the stroke. It was not the same as I had hoped and looked forward to. I was not used to the surroundings. I was fully dependent on everyone- for bathing, toiletries, mobility,

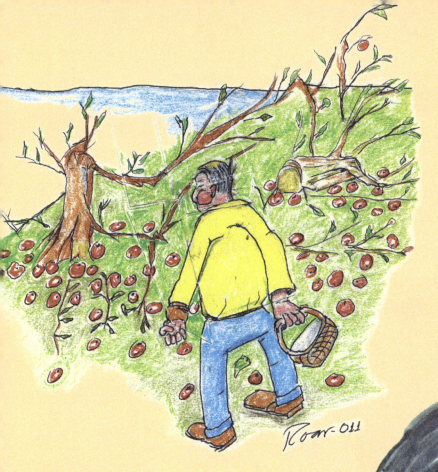

transfers etc. At the hospital, I had doctors, nurses, care aides, rehab and therapists. But at home, I felt I had become a strange person. It was very hard on my family and me.

We renovated the house to suit my physical needs, but it did not suit my spiritual needs. I did not feel at home. This made me unhappy. I did not feel like a Dad. I wanted to find a job that I liked, but the problem was I was trying to get back to life before the stroke. I was trying to live despite the stroke as opposed to living fully within the limits of my physical issues. Recovery had not occurred yet.

Katarina's journal entry:

We tried our best. My mother found herself with the insurmountable and ominous task of looking after all of Roar's needs while she herself was in fragile health. Yes, we brought in home care. Yes, I was there all the time, and so was the rest of the family, but my father required constant care. I do not regret that we tried, but my father's spirit was broken, as was my mother's. Roar became more and more isolated and began to fade.

After one year at home, I arranged for a tour of Evergreen House, the residential care center adjoining the hospital. I collected together information and positive affirmations, and reasons why it was a good move, into a binder and presented it to Roar in his bedroom at home. I will never forget that day. I recall walking up the hill to their home, with binder in my bag and lead in my legs. Thankfully, my father accepted the idea.

The staff at Evergreen House offered the advice to give it six weeks. I would receive tearful, heart-wrenching phone calls from Dad. He would write long letters requesting to come back home. One letter contained only one sentence, *Why am I here?*

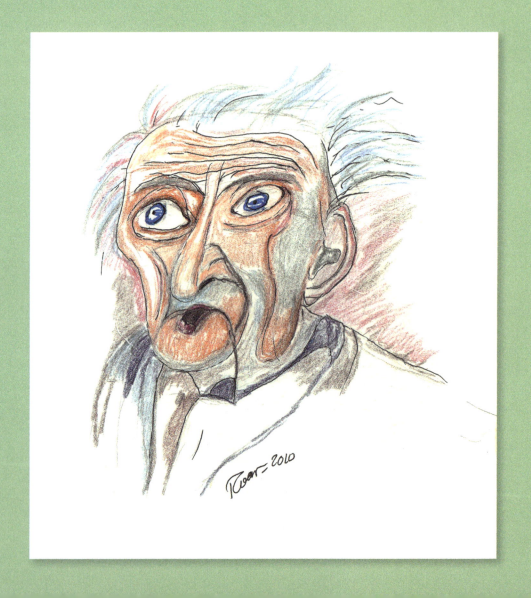

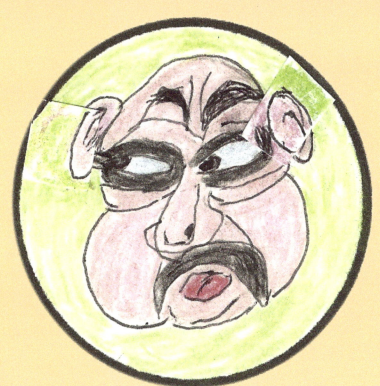

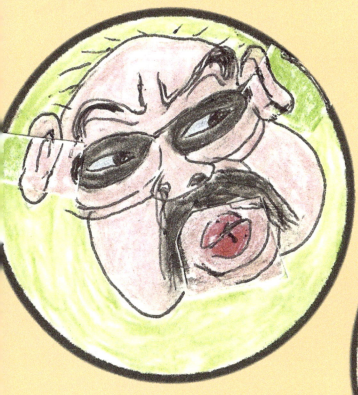

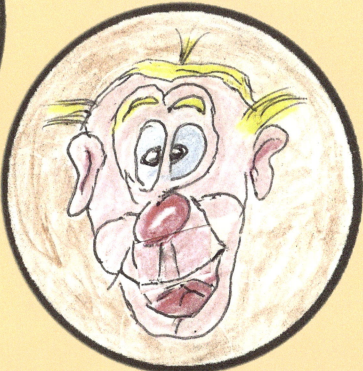

CHAPTER SEVEN: Evergreen House

... to draw one out of the abyss of unbeing.
Marcel Proust

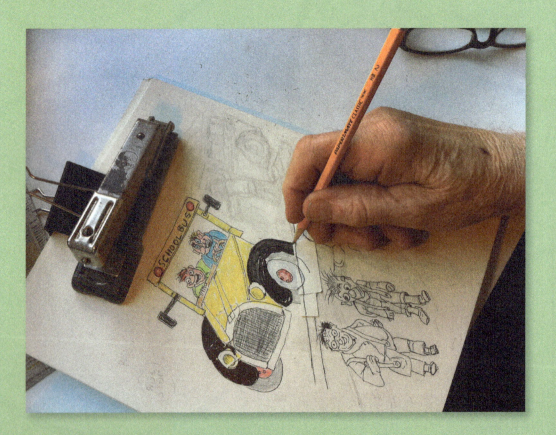

Roar's journal entry:

After one year living at the house, I started to get the feeling that I was a burden. After discussions with the family, I felt that to make it easier for the family, I needed to move into Evergreen. The family agreed that it was best. The atmosphere was similar to rehab and I felt at home but this adjustment was equally strange. *Give it 6 weeks*, the staff said. I installed my super poles, set up my office, set up my new space. This turned out to be the right thing to do. Staff now looked after my physical needs. My room started to become my home. This was mainly thanks to the family and all the nice care aides. I've been in this room since February 2007. When I sit at my desk, I look out over Grouse Mountain.

How the hell am I not depressed now? I'm in diapers, in a wheelchair, with a paralyzed left side and I live in an old age home! Wouldn't it be normal to be depressed? I have a voice and I know what I like and don't like. When I first started living at Evergreen, the nurses would always ask- *why don't you join us in the dining room for mealtimes?*

I tried once for one minute. When I sit in the dining room, I'm sorry, but I cannot stand looking at old people. Yes, I'm old, but who gives a shit? Many families may think it's better for their loved one to be in the dining room, but that's not necessarily true. Most of these people are pushed into the dining room and they just sit at several round tables. When I look around in that big room, I don't want to be reminded that is what I look like that and that is what life could be. I find it depressing and that is why I won't go to the dining room even if they try to force me. It's NOT appetizing to eat there.

In my case, it has nothing to do with age. It's just my own impression. I can never be one of them. I'd shoot myself. The care aides understand. The food isn't great, unfortunately. They said the menu was going to be better. But there's no change. Same old meatloaf. By the way, when my dog is here, I offer him my meatloaf. He sniffs it and walks away. That tells you something! I cannot really eat anything on the menu, but my dog welcomes most of it!

I sometimes write: *to the Chef: thank you for a good meal*, on the menu card. It pays off to be nice! The same goes for all the staff, like the cleaning girls. I regard them all as my friends. The food services personnel are extremely

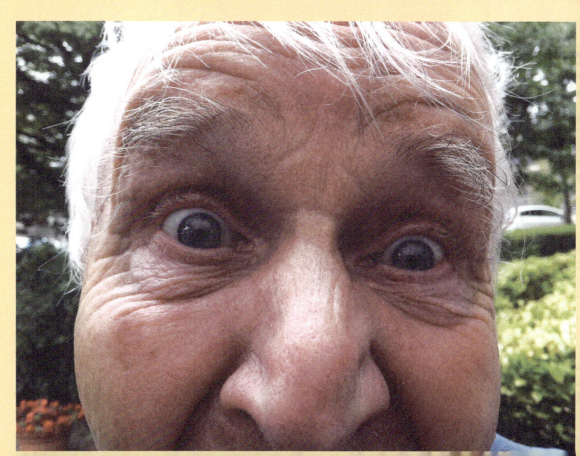

nice, and sometimes I give them a handful of candy. I keep a supply on hand of candy and gum to give to the staff. Treating the staff as friends and giving them treats and lending an ear when they need to sit and chat, creates an atmosphere you want to live in! Don't ever be snotty-faced to people that help you. On the contrary- the nicer you are, the nicer they will be. They are not my servants. They are my friends. By helping them, I help myself. Simple as that.

What do I really need? A shot of whiskey. A cup

of black coffee. My pens and my paper. TV on in the background. A view of Grouse Mountain. That's all I need. Visits with my daughter, petting my dog, working on this book. I have now been in my room for five plus years. Roommates have come and gone. Most of them have died. And the last one will be shot. I'm supposed to be nice, but I can't! I have no patience! And I'm sorry to say, I cannot look forward to being "one of them."

Roommate number one was already in the room when I arrived. He was very quiet. During one funny incident, I was drawing at my desk and I heard a bang. I turned around and I saw two feet sticking up in the air.

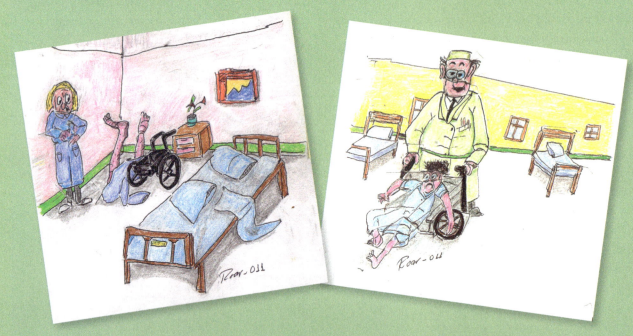

Roommate number two was strange. His background was in medicine. Every second day he had to go to dialysis. He was shouting all the time, and demanding this and that. Once he accused me of being a bad grandpa. I was furious. I wheeled over to get closer to tell him off. But I was so upset, and I was going too fast, I hit the corner of the bed and fell on the floor. He asked if I was OK. I responded with, *go fuck yourself.* He called the nurse!

Towards the end of his life though, he was moved to the transition room. This is where the family goes to say goodbye. Since he was actually my friend, I went in there and told his family, *I'm sorry. He was a good man.* I held his hand. Within a few minutes his hand became cold and he passed away. It was the first time I held a dying person's hand.

Roommate number 3 was probably the biggest guy I have even seen. He was a school principal. He was a friendly guy, but snored like a train! He understood jokes. You could see he was going downhill when he started to just stare instead of eating. He was also moved to the same transition room and spent a couple of weeks there before he died peacefully.

Now I have a new roommate. He may be the strangest person I have ever met. And there have been a lot of strange ones! Let's just leave it at that.

Katarina's journal entry:

It's the fatigue that sets in after a visit that's the hard part. It's the juggling of the schedule, the continuous planning and plotting and moving here and there is a lot of energy output that I don't notice in the moments I am with Roar. But afterwards. It's not grieving, or sentimentality. It's just plain output. And then continuing on to the next role as mother, art therapist, artist, homemaker, pet owner, blogger, youth coordinator, craftivist etc.

I'm my father's daughter. He's often referred to me as his secretary, his boss, his mother, and his wife. But he gets it. And so do I. I'm his daughter. And with that role comes responsibilities. My mother set an example for me as to the level of care and output I should do/ can do/ am capable of.
And I just do it. Because it's like breathing.

As I write this, I am in the midst of a weekend of sticky fatigue and long to do's, but the toolkit is out to remind me that *by letting it go, it all gets done.*

My every-second-day visits are full and busy. Fold the laundry, pack the clean cutlery and Tupperware into the cart, add the clean laundry to the pile, shove in the old envelopes, check if Roar needs any printouts, pack up the car with the dog and computer and journal and purse and sock monkey bag (just in case we watch a video together and I can sew). Head to the grocery store for supplies: Gas-X, Listerine, toothbrush, toothpaste, razors, shaving crème, pens, paper, salami, cheese, grapes, granola bars, gum, chocolate, lollipops, instant coffee, ketchup, blackcurrant jam, air freshener. Pick up a bottle of whiskey, new art supplies, and pizza. Load it into the room. Give the room a good clean. Load in supplies and laundry, fill fridge. Put dirty laundry and orange juice containers (my father saves the extra ones for me) into cart. Grab the envelopes of news clippings he has collected for us. Get Roar ready, pack his messenger bag, head to cafeteria to the favorite table (it must always be the same table), get fresh coffee, ice cream, etc., go through to-do list, get down to work. After a couple of hours, take him back up to his room, unload his stuff, give him the time to check that we didn't forget anything, grab the dog, dirty laundry and hug and kiss goodbye. Ensure his phone is plugged in and routine is adhered to!

Surprises don't work. One-on-one visits are best. Too many people and my father gets flustered. Surprise changes in routine? Avoid. Podiatrist visits are down to a strict choreography. That includes a stop in at Safeway. It works. There is a lot of laughter and humour. And we get each other.

Throughout all this I am lifted by my father's enthusiasm. Despite being wheelchair bound and dependent on care aides for daily needs, he is empowered by art. There have been days when he's called to say he didn't have time for a visit as he had to finish a sketch.

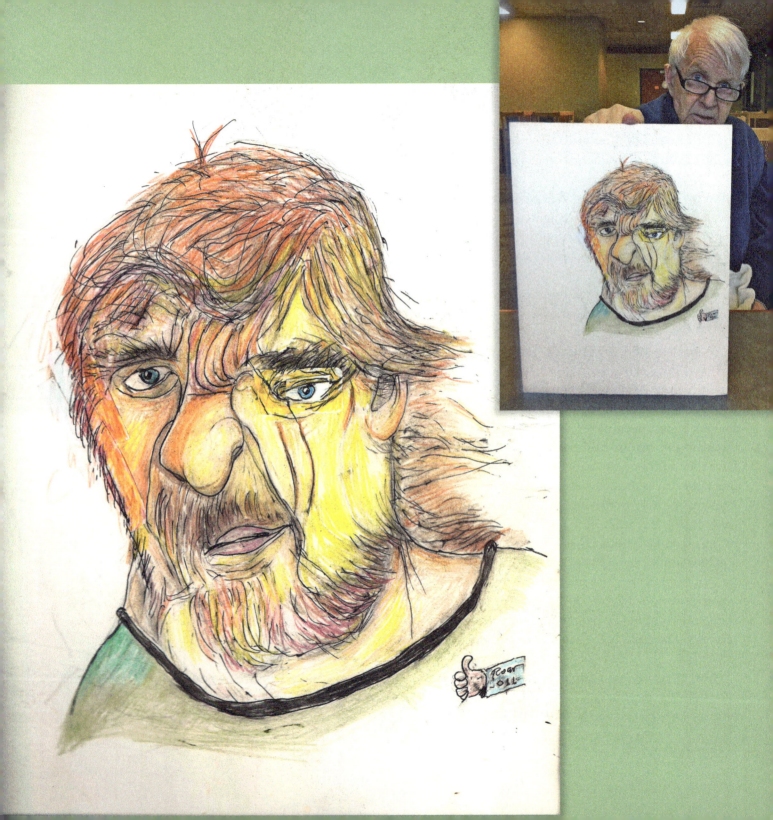

CHAPTER EIGHT: Karin

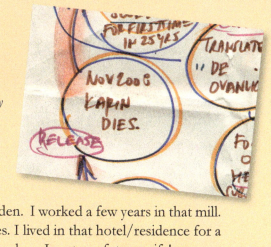

A mother is a person who seeing there are only four pieces of pie for five people, promptly announces she never did care for pie.
Tenneva Jordan

Roar's journal entry:

I started at Skoghallsverken. It was one of the largest mills in Western Sweden. I worked a few years in that mill. Instead of living at a hotel, the mill had a residence and we always had parties. I lived in that hotel/residence for a few years. One day I was invited to one of these residence parties and that's where I met my future wife!

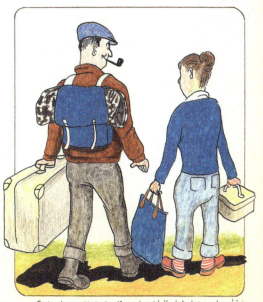

Fredag loaug. kl. 19.30 lämnade vid Karlstad, semestern börjar –.

I would see her around often. She worked at the lab. I met one of Karin's friends. He was kind of snotty, driving around in an Alfa-Romeo. When I saw that car I was irritated. All I had was a bike. I painted it silver. After that everyone called it the *Silver-Arrow*, and that silver bike won over Karin's heart over that Alfa-Romeo.

I was frequently invited for dinner with her parents. Karin's mother was a great cook. Karin and I decided to get married. The marriage was held in Hammarö Church. It's an old wooden church, very well known and popular to get married in. It's just outside of Karlstad.

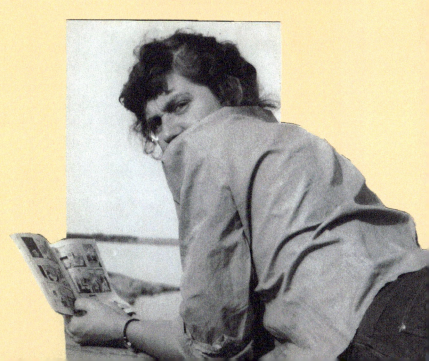

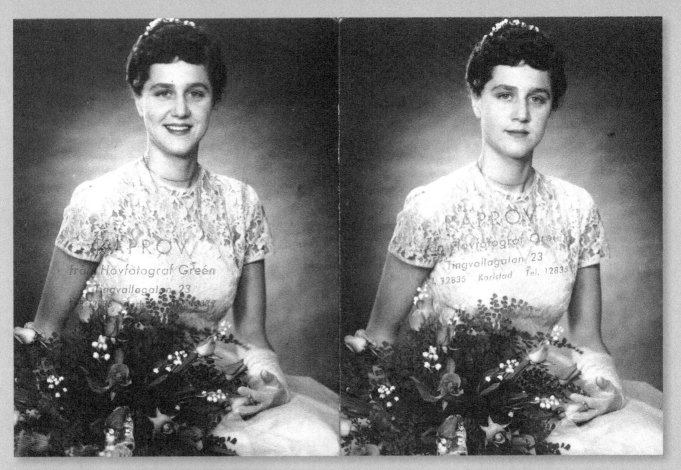

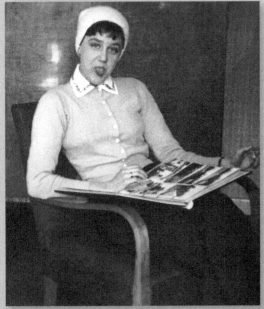

I was used to living in the company hotel but since we were married, we decided to move into a 2-bedroom apartment in Skoghall center. We settled and I bought my first car, an old Mercedes. But it broke down on the way home from the dealer in Karlstad! Everyone laughed. I was advised by friends to get a Volvo and I used it for several years.

After a year, Karin was pregnant. I was offered a job with Billerud in Grums. It was much larger than Skoghall. We started in an apartment block on Ringvägen. We suddenly had tons of friends-Carlssons, Hallgrens, Skååres, and Envalls. We would go to each other's apartments via an underground basement tunnel.

One day, the company general manager visited me. He advised

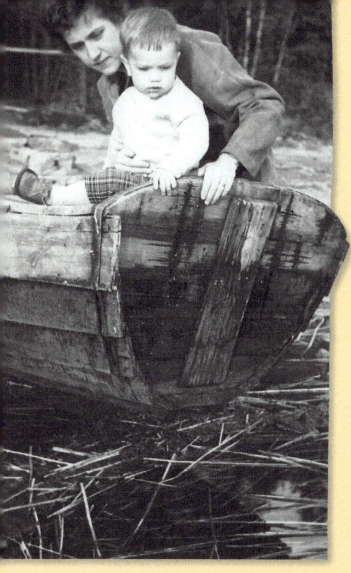

us that they were moving us to a brand new house on Råbäcksgatan. Karin was pregnant again. We eventually had three kids –Anders, Katarina and Fredrik. One couple from Ringvägen became our next-door neighbors when we all moved to houses. Everyone helped each other. It was a beautiful time.

Katarina's journal entry:

I am drenched in memories as I work on this book and find myself obsessively looking at photos of my mother. She's around 20 years old in the photos and just starting her adult life. I love it, but it's also overwhelming, knowing the path that lies ahead of her. I walk in the rain and cry, allowing the grief to present itself. I then let myself process it in my journal.

My mother died after a battle with pancreatic cancer in 2008. Looking at old photos I am struck by Karin's beauty and innocence as she starts her life with my father. I am humbled by the knowledge I have, but she didn't have then, of what lay ahead. I am shattered by the thought that she would lose her mother when she was just age 28. I can't imagine. She was a motherless daughter as she struggled through raising us. She loved so fiercely. She lived! Karin raised her children, as a mother should - with full bellies, clean

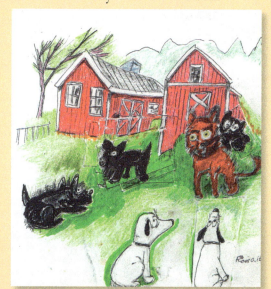

clothes, tons of support and enthusiasm and safety. Yes, with mom, I felt safe. She faced a lot of heartache in her life. She also experienced a lot of joy.

Recently, I took apart my grandmother's old bench to reveal the old cloth and stuffing, daring to look into the interior to face the loss of that time.

This was a grieving exercise as I battled dark feelings and took some precious hours to focus on my mother's absence.

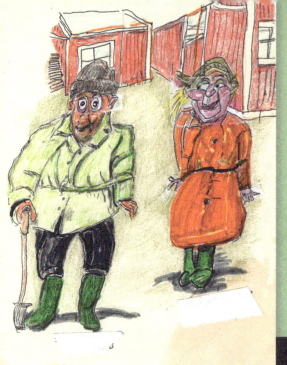

I was raised with that little bench, which sat for years at our summerhouse in Värmland. Its original cloth has remained underneath a myriad of coverings. It is a beautiful worn floral piece that reminds me so much of my grandmother, Stina.

I pulled it apart and found the original stuffing, which unfortunately crumbled in my hands. I wonder what stories were caught up inside all those strands. These are those heartbreaking moments when I realize I can't ask my mother about those stories anymore.

My mother and father certainly loved each other and had a rich life together, but for years they were isolated from each other emotionally. I was a buffer between them all my life. After my mother passed away, I spoke deeply about these issues with my father and it was a gift for both of us to process the past, embrace it and let it go.

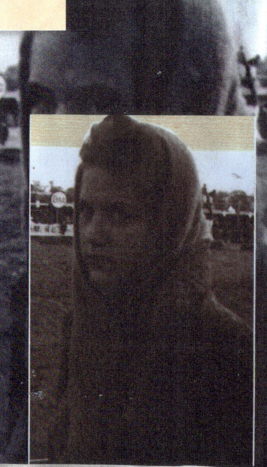

NOV 22, 2010 1:17PM
SOMETIMES YOU HAVE TO STAY
HOME AND CRY. LET ME PICK
UP TWO STEPHEN LEVINE BOOKS
THAT HAVE HELPED ME THROUGH
SOME UNBEARABLE TIMES. WHERE
DOES "WHO CARES?" FALL OPEN
TO? OMG — I JUST WROTE "WHO
CARES?" WHEN THE TITLE IS
"WHO DIES?". [WOW.] IT FALLS
OPEN TO P. 147. "WE ARE EACH
IN A PROCESS OF AWAKENING.
BECOMING FULLY BORN SO THAT
WE MAY DIE EACH MOMENT PAST
OUR FEAR AND ISOLATION. THE
ILLUSION OF SEPARATENESS DIES TO
REVEAL THE DEATHLESSNESS OF
OUR ESSENTIAL NATURE." "A YEAR
TO LIVE" FALLS OPEN TO: P. 68
" AND OFFERING ME HER
SHOULDER SHE WHISPERED, WHEN
A THOUSAND PEOPLE LOOK AT THE MOON
THERE ARE A THOUSAND MOONS."
TODAY I TAKE THE DAY TO RECUPE—
TO DARE TO TAKE CARE OF
MYSELF AS I TAKE CARE OF
MY HOME. I TOOK APART
MORMOR'S (MY MOM'S MOM) OLD
BENCH TO REVEAL THE OLD CLOTH
STUFFING. DARING TO LOOK INTO
THE INTERIOR TO FACE THE LOSS OF
THAT TIME.

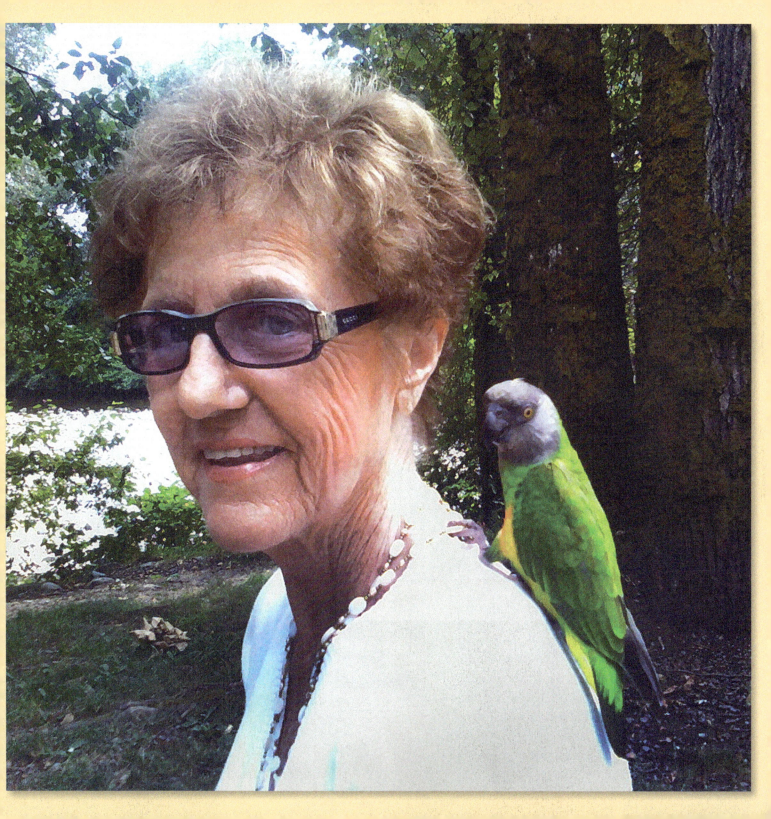

CHAPTER NINE: De Ovanliga

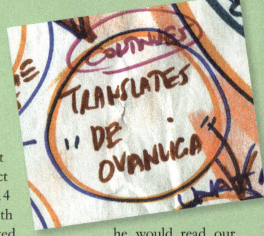

I have had a very rich life and I regret nothing.
Helena Langenhed

Katarina's journal entry:

After my mother passed away, I took my son to Sweden for my first visit in 25 years. It was July 2009. My father celebrated the idea, despite the fact that I would be away for two weeks. I set him up with 14 sets of shorts, 14 t-shirts, 14 pairs of socks and all the supplies he would need. He and I both agreed that I would call whenever possible but in order to stay connected he would read our favorite book, *De Ovanliga*, and immerse himself in Sweden. The book is a delightful photo essay by Åke Mokvist focusing on eccentric Swedish individuals. My mother and father bought it for me during their last trip to Sweden in 2001.

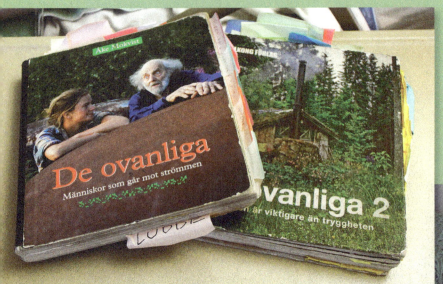

Leaving the book with Roar was the catalyst for eventually creating this book. My father began translating *De Ovanliga* into English while I was away. He said it felt like he was visiting Sweden with me. Actually, while in Sweden, I purchased *De Ovanliga 2* as a special gift to bring home to him.

My father has devoured these books! They are full of post-its, margin notes, coffee spills etc. The day that Roar drew a portrait of Helena Langenhed, who is featured in both books, was the day his current collection of drawings began to build. From July 2009 to present day, Roar has been in full creative process, creating portraits, scenes, and writing words of wisdom.

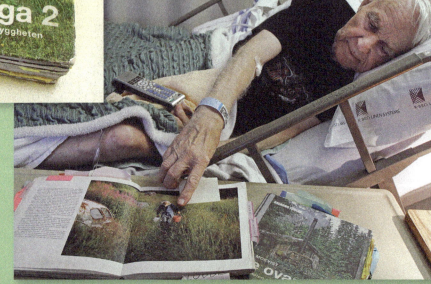

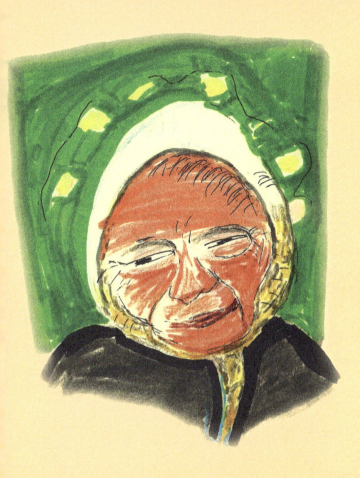

De Ovanliga- människor som går mot strömmen.
The Unusual, only dead fish float with the stream.
Translated from the original Swedish, by Roar Thorsen

Can we really live the way we want to in Sweden? Are all people
valued the same? Or are these just empty political catch phrases and
wishful thinking? Is the strive for wealth, and the hustle and bustle
of daily life, really necessary? Is it not time to re-evaluate? Who
has the highest standard of living? A stressed out city person or a
country philosopher?
…The list of dead originals could be long. But don't you remember
the originals of your childhood? It may be time to reevaluate them!
Many were locked up in mental asylums simply to hide them away
from society and unfortunately the same thing happens today. The
originals are seldom accepted until after death, when we realize their
importance and make radio documentaries, theatre plays, books and
museums about these people.
Åke Mokvist

My father planned to write a script about Helena.

Notes for Rough Draft of Helena, the film, by Roar Thorsen

SCENE: The baptism, October 1917

The story opens with a small farm (*Kopparstad Farm* in Southern Sweden) located in the middle of a large hay field surrounded by a thick forest of spruce and pines. A creek runs across the field past some farm buildings. It runs under the road and into a small lake with a dam before it continues across the field and disappears into the thick forest. A gravel road runs across the field and continues past the small farm. The whole area is peaceful with birdsongs and cows mooing in the distance. The road continues to the neighbouring farm.

Suddenly a horse and carriage, coming out of the forest in a cloud of dust, breaks the silence. Two people sit on the carriage. One is a tall man in black, with hat and white collar. This is the priest Pontén. The other person is a woman dressed in a nurse uniform, the midwife. Inside the carriage two brown leather bags can be seen. Both the priest and the midwife look very serious.

The driver stops in front of the gate to the farm, then continues towards the main building. The carriage stops in front of the building; the priest and the nurse climb out of the carriage and enter into the front porch, carrying their bags. The front door is open; a man and a woman greet both visitors and welcome them in. As they enter they can see into the living room and notice a round table with a stack of towels with a water basin. The ceiling light illuminates up the whole room.

The whole family assembles with the visitors in the kitchen waiting for something to happen. A woman lies in the living room in the bed surrounded by relatives. In the front is the nurse. The midwife asks everyone to leave the room. They all go into the kitchen. After a couple of hours, the guests look at their pocket watches and discuss whether the baby will be a boy or a girl. Suddenly they can hear a baby scream. They all applaud and raise their glasses for a toast, welcoming the baby.

The baby is a good-looking girl with blond hair. The midwife cleans and washes the baby, wrapping her in a blanket. The baby yawns and the midwife gives the baby to the mother. The guests all stand around the bed, admiring the new addition to the Langenhed family. The guests return to the kitchen.

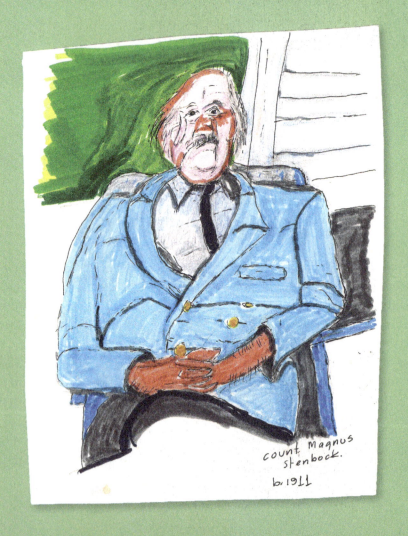

count Magnus
stenbock.
b. 1911

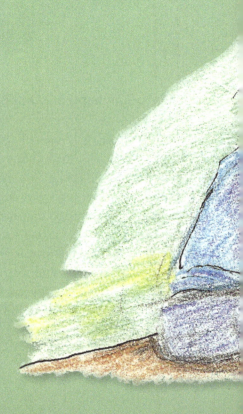

The midwife inspects the baby and says the baby has a weak heart and looks thin. She does not have long to live. The guests come back into the living room, where everything is immaculate ready for baptism- with white crocheted tablecloth and live candles burning. Priest Pontén opens his bible and reads a few lines and recites a prayer. Priest Pontén feels that the baby's name does not matter as she is going to die anyway. But the mother insists.

When the priest pours cold water over the baby's head, the baby girl spits water back straight into his face. The priest says, *I hereby baptize you Helena. May God be with you for the rest of your days.*

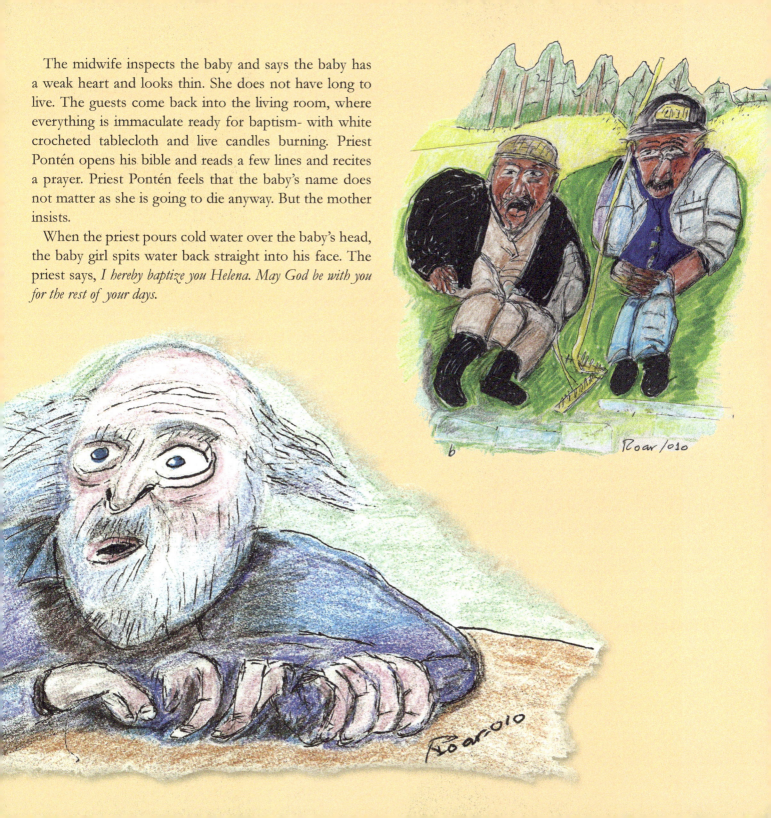

CHAPTER TEN: Cancer

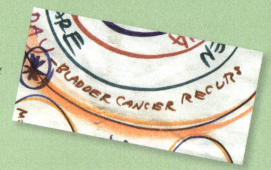

When it came, the wreck left me alive. It flung me on the coast with a warning that what I had to look forward to now was no longer the maximum but the minimum with which I could begin my life afresh… I began to forget what life could not offer and to appreciate what it could…

Frigyes Karinthy

Roar's journal entry:

August 8, 2012 (82nd birthday)

When did the cancer start? Well, at the very beginning, I was working in Meadowlake, Saskatchewan. It was 1996 and I had a meeting with the staff and I noticed during a bathroom break that I was peeing blood. *What the fuck? How do you fix this shit?* I hadn't felt any symptoms. I asked an industrial doctor. He told me to pack my bag and go home to my doctor. So I did. Eventually. After one year. I had to get life insurance and during the urine sample they also noticed blood in my urine. My GP was alarmed. I went for a scope and they discovered a grapefruit size malignant tumor.

The urologist, Dr. Crofts, removed it. It had not penetrated the bladder wall to the muscle so I escaped unharmed. I asked what caused it. He answered, *smoking.* I remember when pipe smoking was not considered smoking on your life insurance policy. My dad and his dad smoked a pipe every day, year round. I was raised on it. I didn't consider it dangerous.

I've gotten many checkups and scopes and more tumor removals over the years. Afterwards, it's always very painful and being wheelchair bound makes it very difficult to recover from scopes. It's difficult to pass the clots. So a few years back I asked to take a break from the exams since I had been clear for several years. I finally had to recheck because I had trouble urinating. The latest scope was in Spring 2012. It showed the cancer had come back. So I went in for the day to remove as much of the tumor as they could and all went well! So far so good! It feels like nothing now. Sometimes I pee a lot, which is normal. The bladder wall is still irritated. But I live with it.

Katarina's journal entry:

September 17, 2012

Sitting in X-ray waiting for my father to have his abdominal X-ray. He's in severe pain and has a bad stomach. Ironically, these are our last few hours of our fundraising campaign for the book. Roar wants to share his journey openly with the world, the blood and guts of life, so I take photos for him. It is the personal he wants to convey. It is just our little story.

September 28, 2012

My body is lead weight. My eyes are swollen. I need to cry, cry and cry. Roar's superpole will be removed in order to make room for the ceiling lift. Have I done enough? Should I have been more aggressive with the scopes way back? I have to remind myself that it was father's choice and his pain and delirium was unbearable after each scope. Instead, he has been able to draw and live his life. What does this mean now, though? I feel heavy, lazy, confused.

I'm sitting at a café and Henrik, my nephew, just woke up and it feels lighter again. We only have these moments. Feeding Henrik banana bread. So how do I work through this apparently *last chapter*? Is that really what this is? What lies ahead? I can't think of that for now. All I really need to do is get through this day. The next five minutes.

October 1, 2012

Sitting in the waiting room as Roar is wheeled into the cystoscopy room. His superpole was removed today. He was upset but accepting. His last claim to independence was in that pole. The staff is supportive, enthusiastic and kind. What happens next? At least this should give some kind of answer? My father is clear as a bell. Is that because of his whiskey and black coffee diet? I'm absolutely overwhelmed, yet also really clear. Why do we hold on so tight to the past and so tight to a perceived future?

Somehow I survived my mother passing and she lives in all of us. She is in me when I hold Henrik, when I live my life. Should I even be anticipating what it would be like to lose my father? That is an anxiety of the heart that may not be beneficial to visit today. I look around the waiting room.

PUSH BUTTON TO ACTIVATE DOOR
RESTRICTED AREA
SCENT-FREE FACILITY
MIXED PAPER

Clock shows 12 noon. About 8 people sit in the wait area some with paper caps waiting their turn.

NO GARBAGE PLEASE
BOUFFANT CAPS, X-LARGE, BLUE
CYSTOSCOPY DISCHARGE INFORMATION
DIRTY LINEN CONTAINER

Cystoscopy confirms bladder cancer is back.

CHECK IN #   EXAM(S)
2078646   80290   CHEST SCAN W/ CONTRAST
                         Ord Diag   ;PULMONARY NODULES, AORTIC ANE

HISTORY: ~~Seizure~~. Pulmonary nodules.

TECHNIQUE: Enhanced helical sections are obtained through the chest.

FINDINGS: This man has multiple bilateral pulmonary nodules, ranging in size from only a few millimeters to up to 3 cm. This is almost certainly due to metastatic disease. There is no evidence of any adenopathy within the chest. No pleural effusion. Small pericardial effusion is present.

No definite sinister skeletal pathology.

With regards to the primary, this is still not entirely established on the basis of this CT scan. I suppose one of the nodules within the lungs could be the primary and the others could be hematogenous metastases. The largest and most dominant nodule is in the right lower lobe and contains a few internal air bronchograms. In the absence of other sites for potential tissue diagnosis, it would be feasible to perform a biopsy of this dominant nodule in the right lower lobe under either fluoroscopic or CT guidance.

COMPUTED TOMOGRAPHY DEPARTMENT

October 5, 2012

Roar's CT scan reveals … *multiple bilateral pulmonary nodules… almost certainly due to metastatic disease…*
I had meeting with the doctor today. She and I then revealed the results to Roar. This brings up a lot of memories around my mother. I have to say, though, it is not scary. I have no unfinished business with my father, just *wish business.*
I'm sitting in the sun at the hospital cafeteria while my father naps and Tobey is playing in the bushes off-leash. I treated myself to a scarf for $20. It's stupid therapy but it's what I needed right now. I must have bought dozens of scarves from the gift shop since Dad's stroke and Mom's treatments. Amazing what a rectangular piece of cloth can do. Time to head back for an evening session with Dad.

October 11, 2012

I was so happy that Roar had a chance to meet with Julie Salisbury, our publisher, today for the first time. Despite his excruciating pain, he had a chance to get to know her and Julie got a hint of my father's infamous and vigorous spirit. Afterwards, Roar and I spent the evening in the emergency to replace his catheter. We watched the debate and laughed and talked about life. Amazingly, it has been 7 years minus one day since Roar made his first post stroke drawing.

October 13, 2012

My father is dying. I accept it. He unwinds before me. I let him go. But losing my best friend is more painful than I anticipated. I fear my heart may cave in on itself. But how can it, when it is so full of love? I don't believe a daughter can love her father more. Knowing that he loves me as much as I do him will carry me for the rest of my life. I sit peacefully sewing sock monkeys and writing by his bed, *Pappa* watching Mr. Bean with a sleeping Tobey beside him.

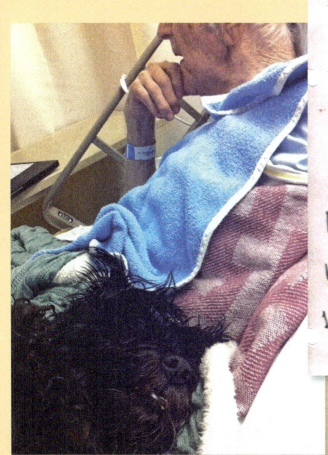

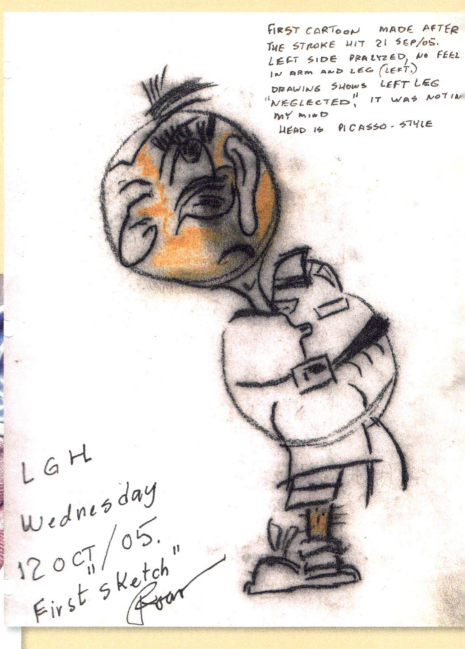

FIRST CARTOON MADE AFTER THE STROKE HIT 21 SEP/05. LEFT SIDE PRALYZED, NO FEEL IN ARM AND LEG (LEFT.) DRAWING SHOWS LEFT LEG "NEGLECTED," IT WAS NOT IN MY MIND
HEAD IS PICASSO - STYLE

LGH
Wednesday
12 OCT/05.
"First sketch"

(25)

W s p a ... d ... d i d
s ... ing 4p ... c l ... ... a
... th ... il was ... e ... ... d ... ne
... ioh ... a c ... me a a ... e ... ... a
... 7t was ... ll No ...
... d book ... at
... an con t ...

GALLERY

I am impelled, not to squeak like a grateful and apologetic mouse, but to roar like a lion out of pride in my profession.
John Steinbeck

Roar's journal entry:

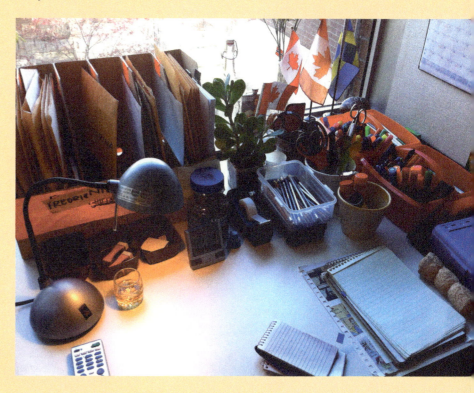

I was very skeptical in the beginning moving in to care, since I had never experienced such a type of life. I learned quickly that the only way to live here was to adjust myself. One of the best things is that all the nurses and staff are incredible and keep me from going insane! I have a wonderful life with all my caretakers and I consider them my daughters (and sons). In addition to all this, I have found a perfect place to do my art.

My previous work consisted mainly of oil paintings and ink drawings. After I moved into Evergreen House, because of space issues, I concentrated on smaller work such as cartoons. I started collecting illustrations for a potential book as a special project with my daughter and indeed, you are holding this book right now.

You may notice my drawings have layers of stickers on them. Many times when I am creating, any mistake makes me think, *I've got to fix this now. I don't like this one. My mistake, start again.* But how do you erase a mistake that is in ink? When it is necessary to erase ink drawings, my simple solution is to use white stickers. Covering the mistakes, I can continue with the basic idea. The drawings are given new shape. A typical cover-up!

Express yourself. Nobody else has advantage over you. Your thoughts are your own. They are you. What do you want to do? How? With what? What pen? On what? You converse with yourself. Should I use black ink? Color? Paint? Pens? Crayons? Colored pencils?

During the day I make my own sketches based upon inspiration from comics and newspapers, books etc. At the end of the day, I hang the pictures on the wall across from the foot of my bed. I self-criticize, critique, analyze, question. I start again the next morning. *That looks better.* I repeat this the next day. It takes forever as an artist to approve a project. *Nose wrong. Ears wrong.* Corrections never stop until you are satisfied. Hopefully this attitude keeps you on track. Keep making it better. That is the artistic process. The advantage is that you do it the way you think it should look like. You always keep in mind: *it could be better*.

What motivated Rembrandt and everyone else? What makes artists do amazing work? I know Van Gogh never liked his own work. Maybe if you go too deep into art, it hurts you. You can never tell an artist what to do. Everything has to come from your own heart and brain.

Art makes you happy and patient. Making a drawing takes a long time. I find inspiration concentrating alone, being calm and undisturbed. A drawing is your thoughts on paper. I sit at my desk in a residential care center, which gives me the possibility to work all day. It also gives me the freedom to create what I like. I never thought that making a drawing in a rest home would give me any inspiration. Actually I am scared that I have so much fun creating anything that I want. Sitting alone at my table gives me the freedom to do what I like without criticism. Art is cheap. All you need is inspiration. A couple of pencils. A table. And a single chair.

GALLERY:

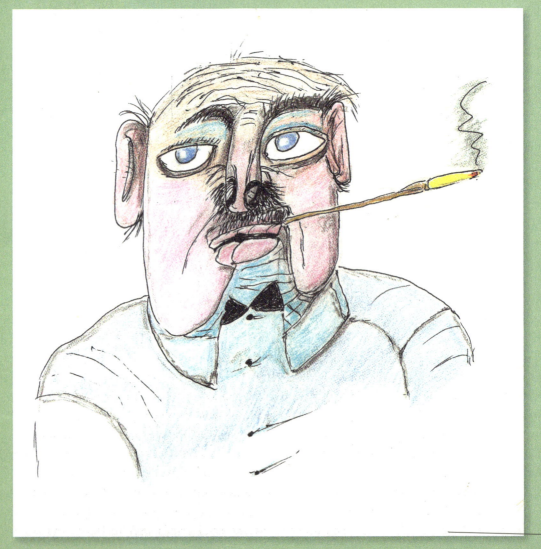

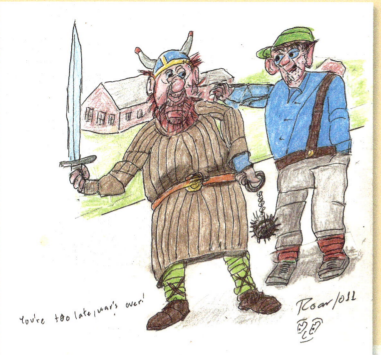

You're too late, war's over!

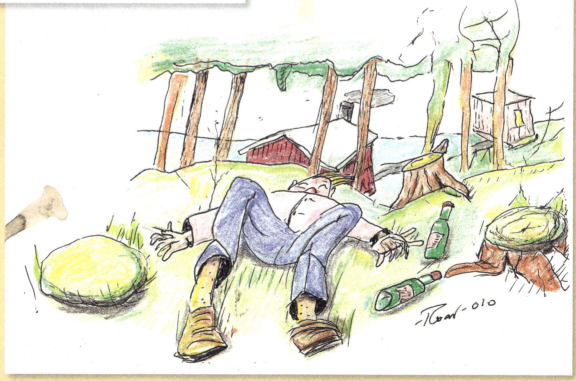

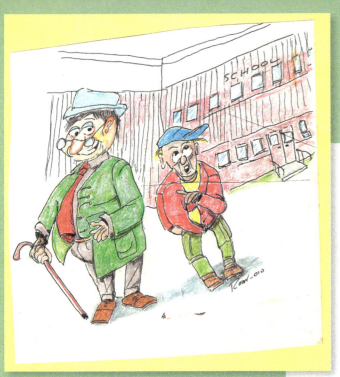
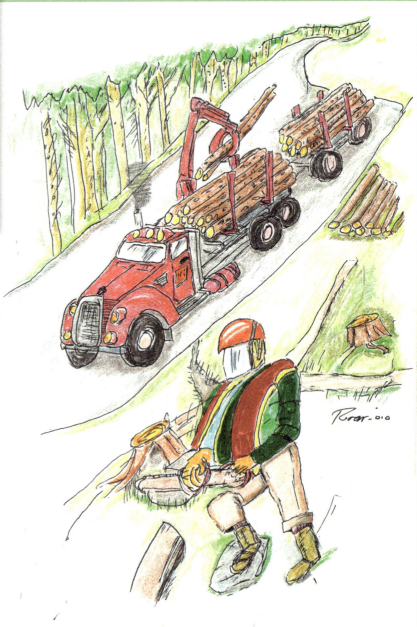

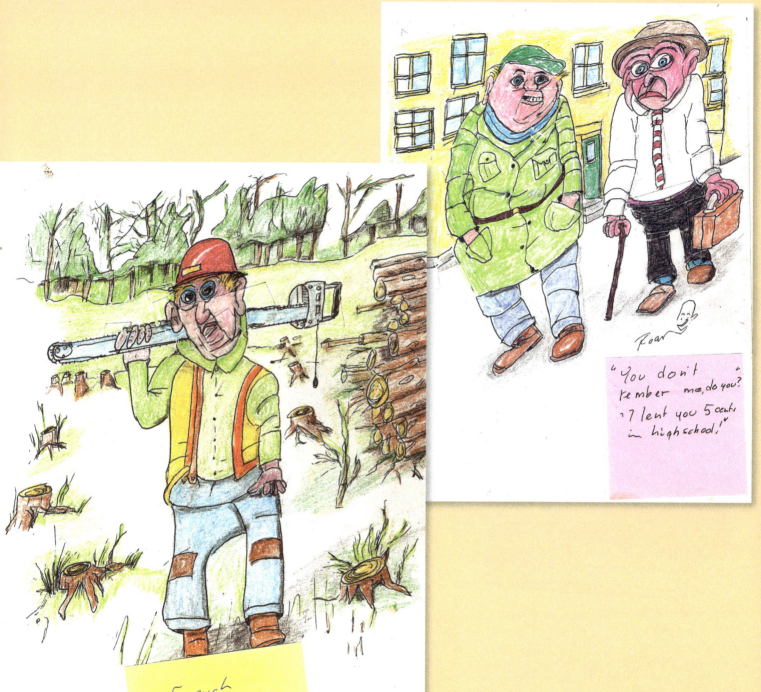

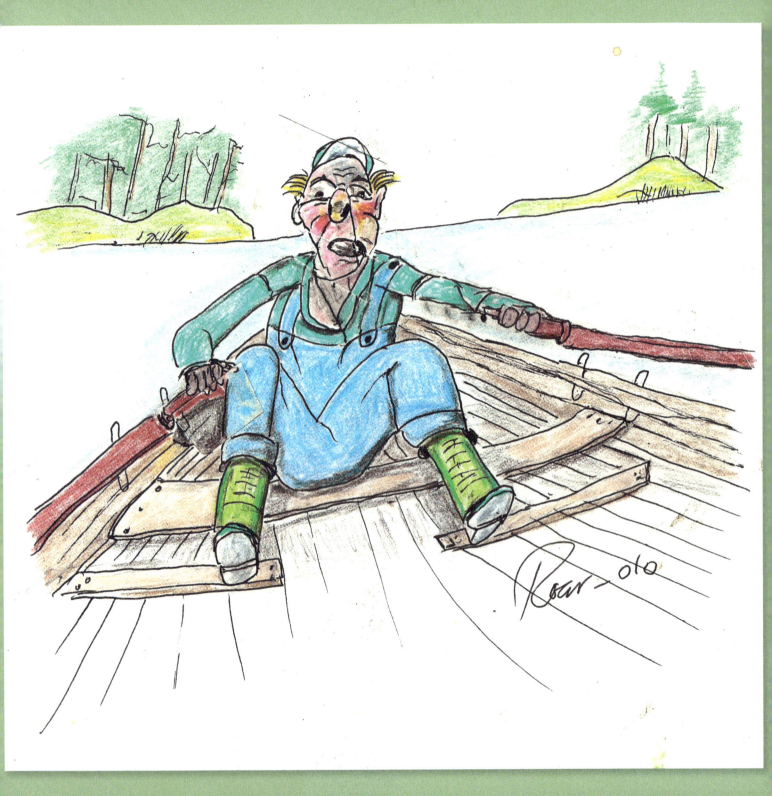

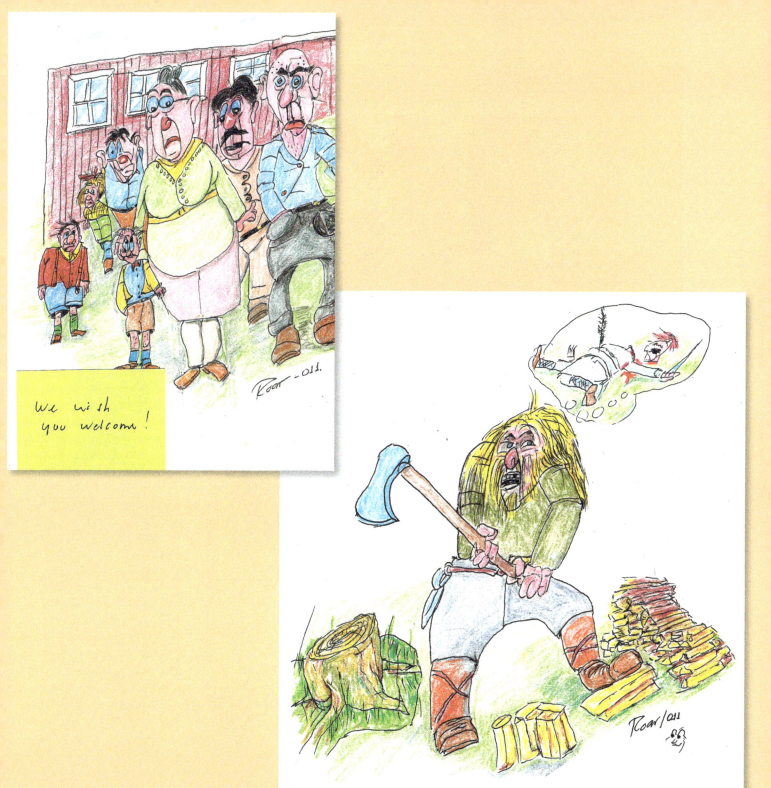

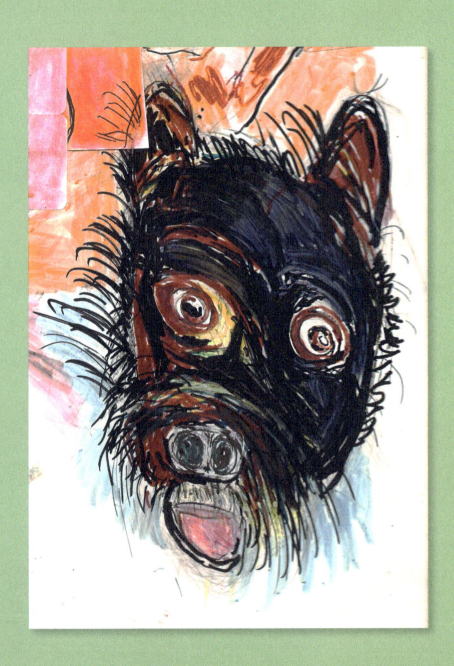

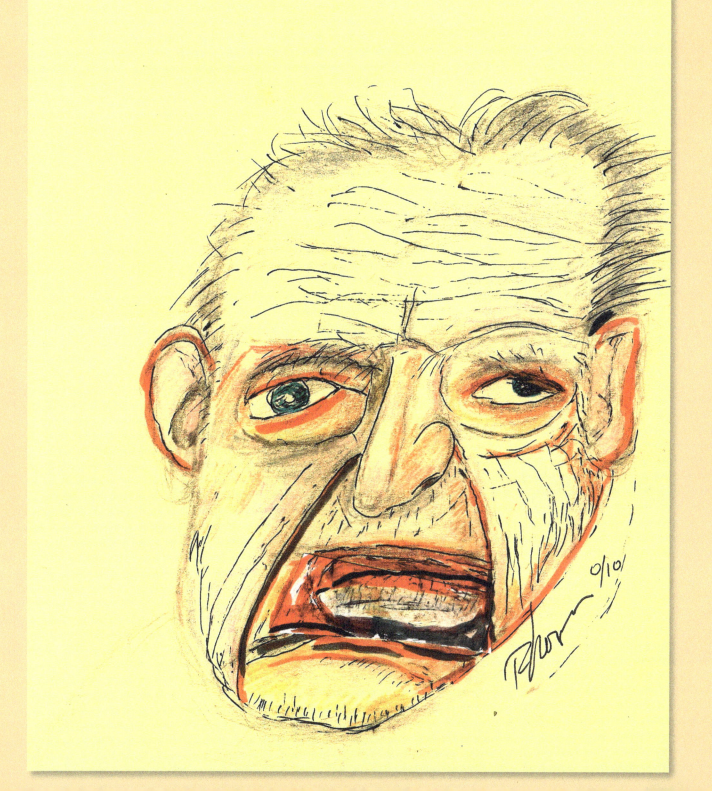

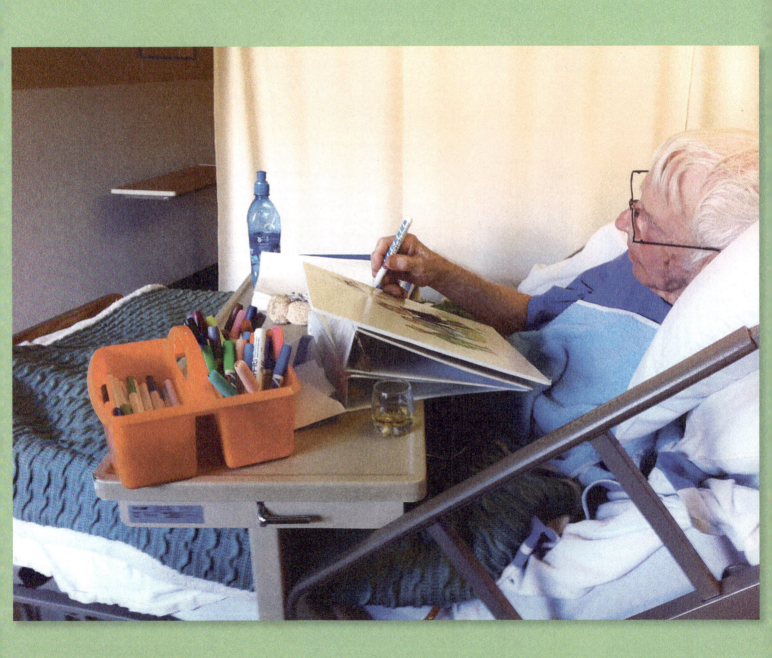

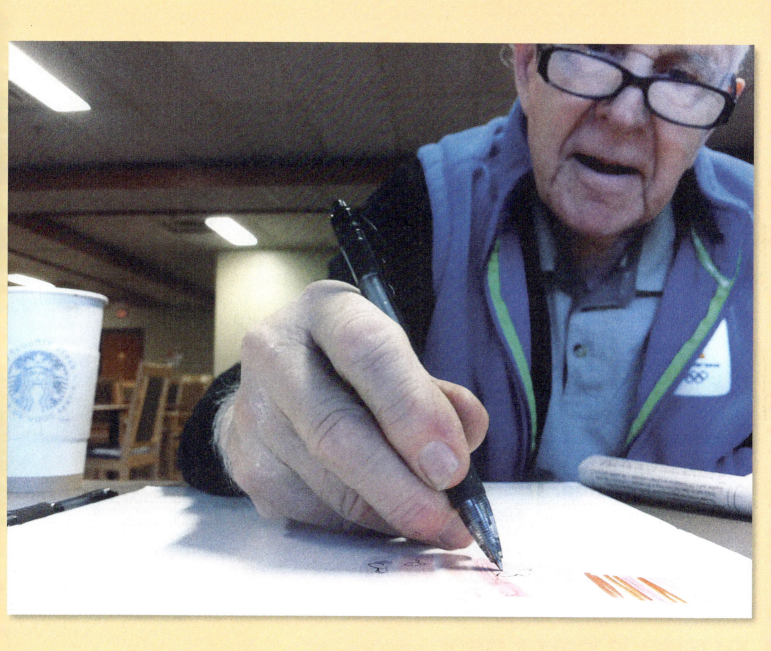

EPILOGUE

After his last scope on October 5, 2012, that showed a predictable recurrence of his bladder cancer, I watched my father excitedly get back to his desk and get back to work. But alas, he became bed-ridden the following day.

As fatigue and pain took over, Roar mourned the loss of being able to draw, yet he enjoyed looking at the drawings on his wall and petting his dog, Tobey. We would reminisce about the journey we took together and our connection through art.

On October 19, 2012, I had to make a major decision. Do I agree to let my father undergo bladder surgery despite his deteriorating condition or say no? The doctor claimed he had a fighting chance. I felt an anxiety building in my gut. Something didn't seem right.

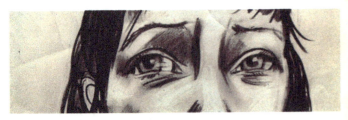

ART HEALS

Jan 21- Feb 7, 2012

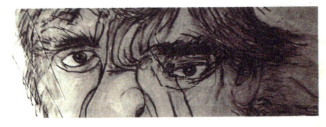

Therapeutic art by
Katarina and Roar Thorsen

RUBBLE GALLERY
1879 POWELL ST
opening ART EVENT
Jan 21 7-9 PM

When I saw Roar on the transport stretcher, unresponsive and in pain, I said *no* to the surgery and asked for his immediate transfer back to his room. There were hugs from the nurses and tears of agreement. The care aides at Evergreen also cried with relief when we got back. They gently placed him back in his bed, washed him and tended to him.

For a week, we remained at Roar's bedside. For the most part, my father was peaceful; his medication doses were increased daily in order to prevent breakthrough pain. He slept soundly with a strong heartbeat. He would reach out once in awhile to people and things we could not see and

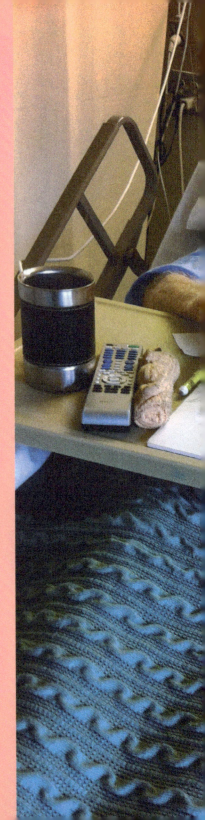

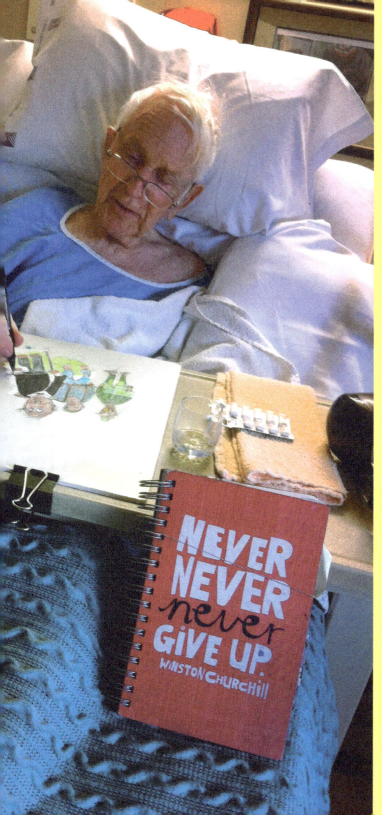

make surprising sounds of recognition when staff would come in.

We became gypsies– a family in need to set up camp, to support each other and to surround our father with love and the sounds of life.

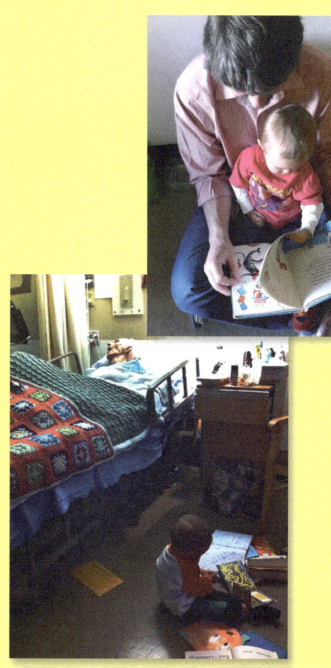

We were not so much waiting to be with Roar at the moment he let out that last breath, as much as we were showing him that we are living, laughing, loving, moving into our future by expressing our gratitude through our presence. It was also an opportunity to bond as a family and re-process losing our mother in November 2008.

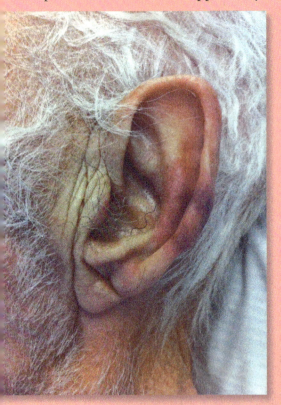

I have cried a lot and I expect to cry a lot more. I anticipate intense missing, but that week I laughed a lot– laughed at my little family as we maintained our camp and cocooned ourselves in room 207 from morning to evening. At the end of the day, we would turn off the lights except for the Christmas lights and the diffuser. The staff would visit Roar all night, and we were happy allowing them their time to show their love and gratitude to him.

Throughout the week my father was working. I could tell. Deep internal work as he let go of his physical body. His eyes remain closed for most of the day. His color remained good.

I came up early in the morning on October 25, 2012 and spent some hours by myself with Roar before the rest of the family arrived for our daily vigil. I set up the space. I had an intense need to offer some kind of guidance for him. I played the *Tibetan book of the Dead- the Great Liberation* video on my laptop, turning the volume to maximum. We were not interrupted and it was very powerful. I played him Swedish lullabies into his left ear.

The family eventually arrived and we spent another beautiful day together.

The staff came in regularly to tend him and to check in. The doctor felt Roar could hang on another two weeks. I was confused, as it did not feel right intuitively. I felt a panic well up. I did not want my father to suffer any more.

We had some family discussion and then packed up around 8:30 PM, turned off the lights except for the Christmas lights and diffuser. Roar was peaceful and apparently pain-free. I sensed he needed time to concentrate and to complete the journey on his own.

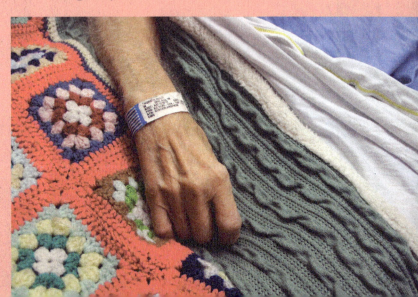

Fifteen minutes after we left, care aide Kim went in and checked on him. He was still breathing. Care aide Mike went in shortly after that and discovered that Roar had finally stopped breathing. I received the call as my son and I bit into our dinner. We quickly headed back to Evergreen. As we walked into the room, we saw that his beloved caregivers surrounded Roar. They had tended him so beautifully.

My son, my brothers, sister-in-law and I sat in the room for an hour talking, laughing, sighing, breathing, planning and sharing shots of Roar's whiskey in his honor. Tobey lay on my father's legs as we awaited the transfer of his body.

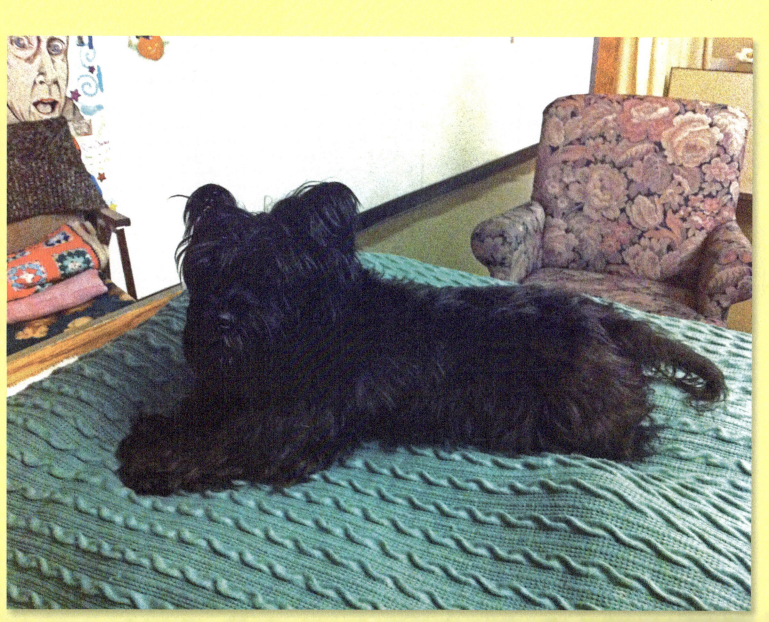

The following day we emptied Roar's room. I am struck by the image of a room filled with life and the stark contrast of a life passed.

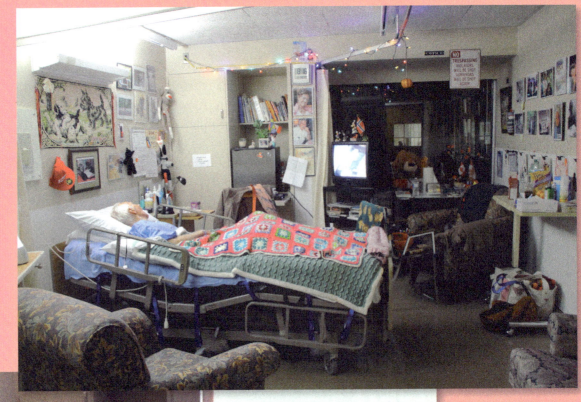

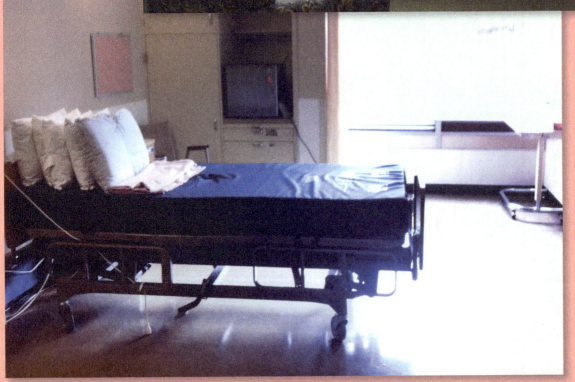

I am filled with joy, relief, love, sadness and all the beautiful emotions a daughter can feel losing her beloved father. I have also lost my best friend and I sense that once the numbness wears off, I will experience intense loss in this regard, but I accept and welcome it for I am so lucky to have had such a friendship.

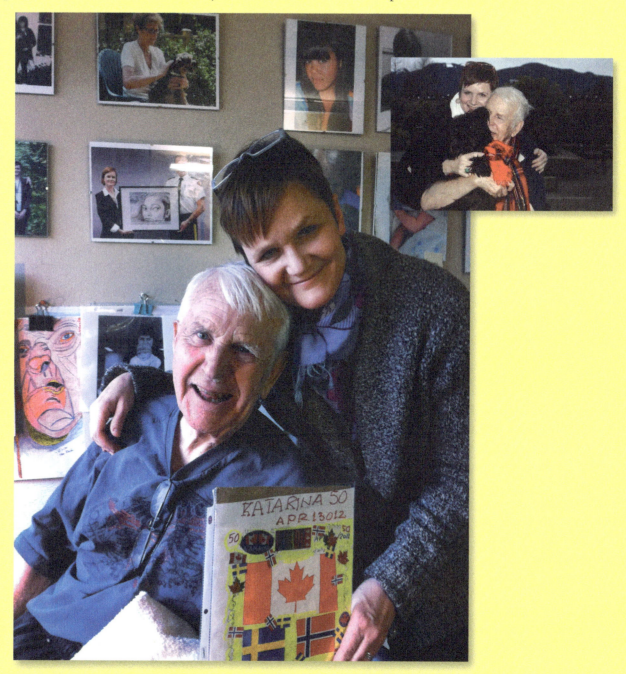

I know that art doesn't cure but it is a powerful tool to facilitate healing. I am truly blessed to witness this healing power of art every day in my work and it is obvious that it helped my father thrive. Art gave him purpose, routine and passion. It helped him reclaim his emotional life. Art met Roar's most fundamental needs: to be fed, to be loved and to be heard. What can be greater than that?

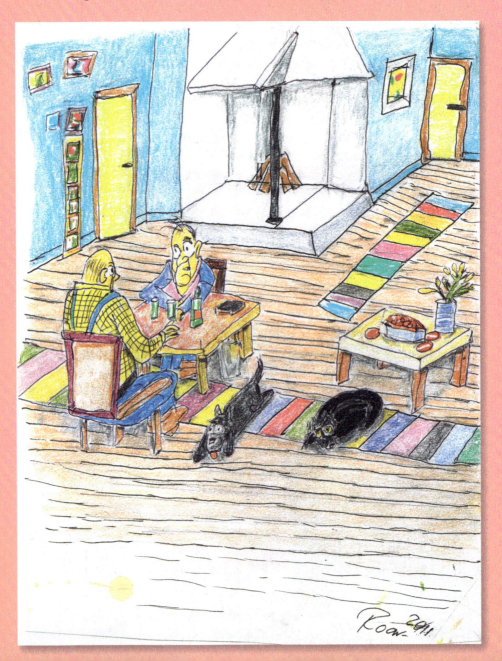

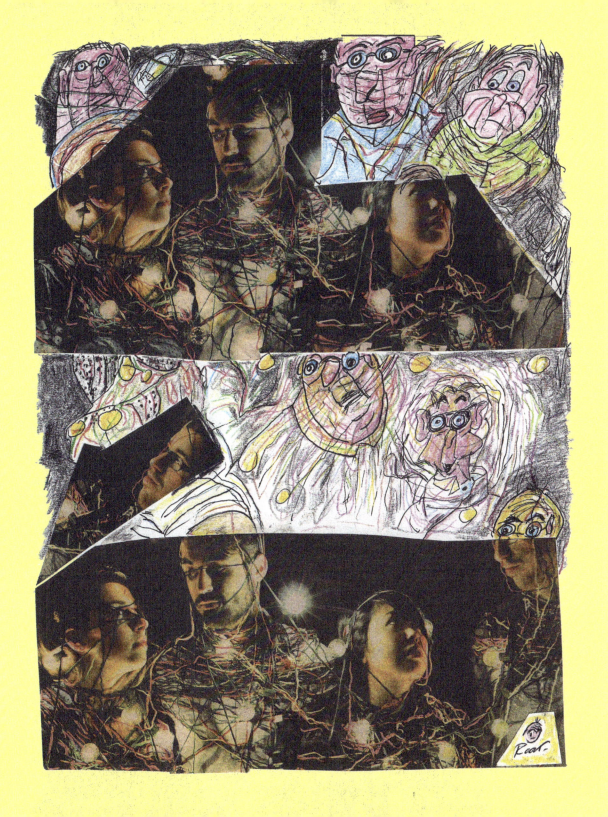

AFTERWORD

We are here to laugh at the odds and live our lives so well that Death will tremble to take us.
Charles Bukowski

Katarina's journal entry:

What has survived in my father, despite any health setbacks, is his spirit and his spirit is what has infused me with the energy to live my own life creatively and fully. Our book is about art and a father/daughter story, but it is also a legacy that we are creating for Roar's grandchildren Anna age 27, Julian age 24 and little Henrik, age 1. My father chose to end this book in two ways, firstly, with letters to his grandchildren and secondly, with a message to the reader.

Note that in Swedish, my father is Anna and Julian's *Morfar* (mother's father) and Henrik's *Farfar* (father's father).

Letters from Roar:

Dear Anna,

What the hell are you doing in San Francisco? Are you OK? Do you want Morfar to come down to help? I could have written this a bunch of years ago but I never thought my little girl would end up there, a long way from Vancouver and think of all the houses you used to live in!

I am very, very proud of my little girl. You sure have come a long way! As always, you can do everything you want! As Morfar always says, *never take no for an answer.* Just kick the hell out of them!

Your mom, Katarina, is very proud of you. And so is Morfar. It is nice that you have so many friends. Sounds safe with all the bodyguards.

Anna, did you hear me? I think you don't have a clue what a nice life you are leading and you did it all on your own! How much money are you making? Sorry, just a joke!

Good luck Anna! Never stop!

Say hi to all your friends. Hope they are happy with helping you!! See you!

Love, Morfar

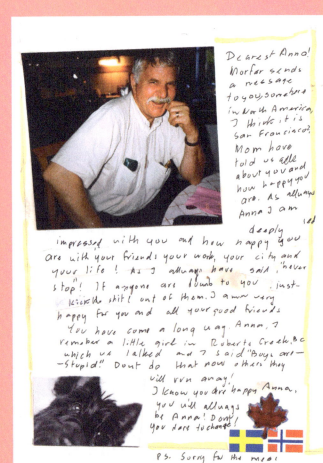

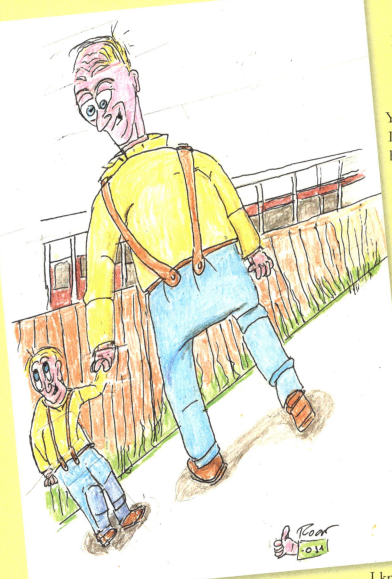

Dear Julian,

Morfar wants to have a word with you.

I hardly need to say it, I am impressed with you. You have come a long way and I really admire you. It's amazing to think back to when you were a little boy on West 4th. In fact, the talk we had together the other day was very good because it just shows the kind of guy you have become. I must say, that I am very proud of you, especially for all the things you have gone through.

Even during the darkest days, you have always kept on going. Most impressive is the way you handle yourself when talking with others. I must admire you very much. I know you have gone through hard times, which is very unique. I don't know how many people realize the various situations in which you have handled yourself so well.

As a matter fact, maybe you are growing too fast! You are quickly becoming famous so I really admire you, Julian! I am sure you are going to do very well in your upcoming life. Never look back. You have a huge life waiting in front of you.

What really impresses me is that you've done all this yourself; you've gone from a shy little boy to becoming a musician with new friends and a whole new life. After all I have told you, I know you can go far. As I told Anna, never stop with what you are doing.

I wish you all the best in your future, Julian. Keep on going! New adventures are just around the corner! Don't forget,you are best yourself. Do not change. As you look forward, you will realize that nothing is impossible. I know that Mom and Anna are very impressed with you. You will notice that the more you work, the more you like it and the more fun it will be. I'm looking forward to listening to all your ideas.

You are also lucky that you have such an amazing mom and sister. All of you are inspirations for each other and because of your good family, I know that you will always succeed. Never give up. If you see a closed door, kick it in. I will always follow your development. So, good luck, Julian. Morfar will count on you! Remember, you are the best.

Love, Morfar

Dear Henrik,

The angel has arrived. One year ago, the Thorsen family expanded to one more boy. Nature is amazing. Farfar is so proud of our new family member! Although you are small and short, you already have an attitude with your amazing smile and blue/brown eyes. I've got a feeling that we are looking upon the *new boss* in the Thorsen family.

Life is amazing. When looking at you, a little angel, I realize the Thorsen family is moving forward. I remember the first time I saw you; you did not have to say anything because I knew we had an instant super member of the family. I recall you as a tiny little boy and now suddenly, you are one year old!

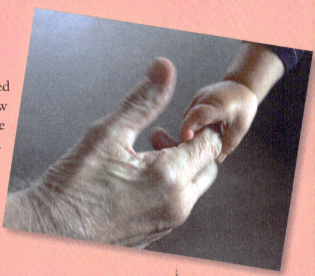

You have made a space for yourself, which is very smart, since no one can say no to a person like Henrik! I envy you, Henrik, for the future is in front of you. Every day will be incredible as you leap forward into your life.

Although you don't know yet what will happen in the future, you have already given a gift to your Mom and Dad, and this gift has quickly turned from a baby to a growing boy. I'm very impressed of God's creation. I look forward to working with you and the family.

Growing up today is not the same as it was for Farfar. As you start your *long* life, you will be happy for every day you are growing up and living *your own life*. Looking at pictures of you, I can already see that you are going to be a very happy boy, which will make your parents happy and proud. You have a long way to go, but you will find out that the future will be an adventure.

You will find out that life has its ups and downs, and you will also learn how to handle all the situations that lie in front of you. Each day will give you a new experience. It will be up to you to ride out the storms. Do not forget: the future is up to you.

As you go through life, you will learn from your parents, family and your future friends. You will find out that life can be both complicated *and* happy.

Love, Farfar

Dear reader,

Stephen Levine wrote: *gratitude is the highest form of acceptance… thankful to be born into this world of shit and sunshine.* I agree. I leave you with three words. *HUMOUR IS MEDICINE.*

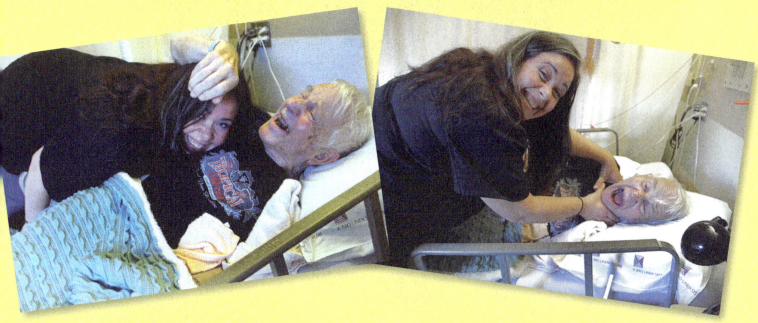

Humour is a lifesaver and it has helped me in every situation. I recall the day my daughter accompanied me to a cystoscopy. I was on the stretcher. We saw the morgue sign and we had an idea. We returned later and took a photo:

It perfectly illustrates my attitude. I put the photo in a frame as a present for the staff room. The care aides and nurses loved it. They squealed with laughter. They put it up on the wall. They said it was the best picture they had ever seen. It says everything. Then all of a sudden, one day, it was returned to me. The supervisor had told them it was not appropriate. Now it hangs on the wall in my room. The care aides and nurses still love it. They still squeal with laughter.

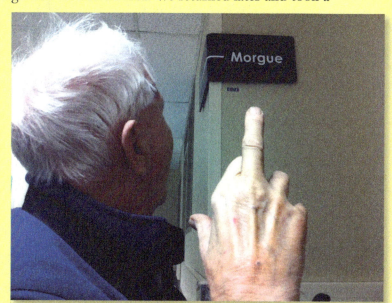

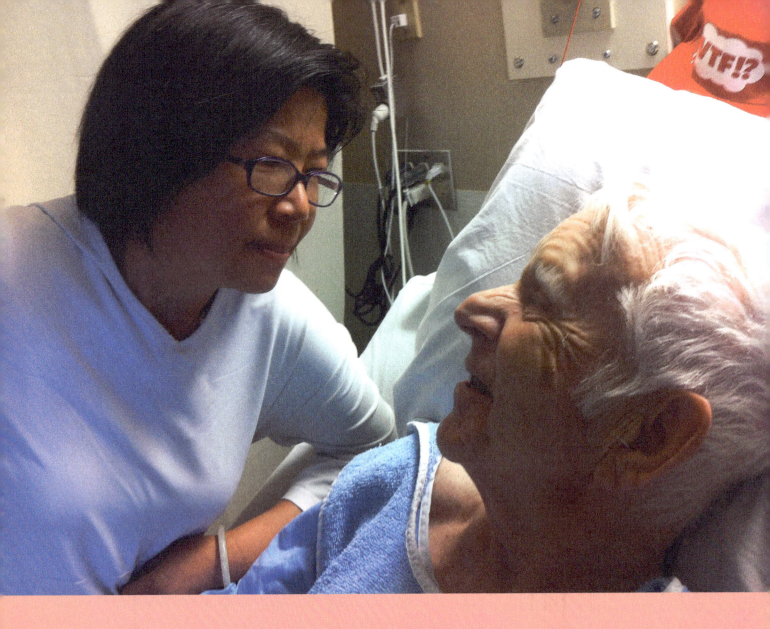

My care aides get it and play along with me. It makes life bearable and wonderful! Never forget that! Never forget to laugh! *HUMOUR IS MEDICINE.*
    Sincerely, Roar Thorsen

AUTHOR BIOGRAPHY

Katarina Thorsen was born in Karlstad, Sweden. She initially came to Canada in 1968, moving back and forth between the two countries until finally settling in North Vancouver with her parents and siblings in 1977. Katarina received a Bachelor of Science (in Biological Sciences) from the University of British Columbia in 1984 and attended Emily Carr College of Art and Design from 1986 to 1990.

Katarina raised two children while pursuing her visual art career and professional development. Her post-graduate studies include fine arts, psychology, special education (focusing on autism, behavioral challenges and juvenile justice), behavioral evidence analysis (criminal profiling) and restorative justice.

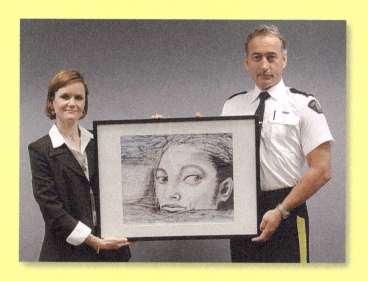

Katarina donated many pieces of artwork in support of Vancouver's Missing Women's Legacy Society. In 2002, she presented the Coquiltam RCMP detachment with a print of *Sarah, I Think of You*, in honor of the victims of Robert Pickton. In 2005, Katarina worked with the Vancouver chapter of Circles of Support and Accountability (community support for high risk sex offenders) and she was the art therapist at Burnaby Youth Custody Centre from 2006 to 2008. Katarina moved on to become the full-time art therapist at Keith Lynn Alternative Secondary School from 2008 to 2011. In 2010, Katarina received the City of North Vancouver's Civic Youth Award: Outstanding Supporter of Youth.

Katarina specializes in providing therapeutic art and outreach support to at-risk youth with a variety of issues including behavioral challenges, learning disabilities, substance abuse and mental health. She currently works on the Downtown Eastside. The goal of Katarina's therapeutic art is to raise self-esteem and facilitate empowerment while developing self-advocacy skills in the client.

Katarina's art classes include painting, drawing, quilting, graffiti, art history, photography, animation, watercolor tattooing and sock monkey therapy. She also provides at-risk youth with skills-training in arts and crafts and the opportunity to sell their work as a source of income.

Katarina's own artwork (drawing, painting, street art, journaling and crafting) can be found in private collections in Canada, United States and Sweden and on the streets of North America and Europe. Her popular interactive art events encourage participants to add to the artwork and become part of the creative process. She is passionate about the therapeutic power of art and its ability to build connections.

Katarina's next book is a graphic novel based on her research into a historical Vancouver murder mystery.

You connect with Katarina at the following sites:

WEBSITE: kat-art.ca
ART BLOG: katthorsen.wordpress.com
CRAFT BLOG: poststreet.wordpress.com
ART THERAPY BLOG: klasssockmonkey.wordpress.com
ETSY SHOP: etsy.com/shop/katarinathorsen
TWITTER: KatThorsen
FACEBOOK: Kat Thorsen
INSTAGRAM: poststreet

View the documentary:
Drawn Together: Roar Thorsen's Recovery Through Art
9:03
Directed, edited, filmed by Julian Bowers
Music by J. Lastoria and Julian Bowers
http://youtu.be/_Pb5a1GPtuQ

A CALL TO ACTION

Choose one or all of the following options:

- Demystify residential care.
- Thank a care aide.
- Become knowledgeable about stroke and cancer risks.
- Journal.
- Laugh a lot.
- Make time, real quality time.
- Gather materials, instruments, inspirations, music, images and all sorts of supplies.
- Start asking questions.
- Start collecting.
- Start connecting.
- Start listening.
- Start facilitating.
- Start creating.
- Recognize your limits and expand within them.
- Celebrate the human spirit.
- Live like you have only one year to live.

If you would like to consult with Katarina regarding facilitating therapeutic art and creative expression in yourself and others, visit her website at katthorsen.wordpress.com

If you want to get on the path to be a published author
by Influence Publishing please go to
www.InspireABook.com

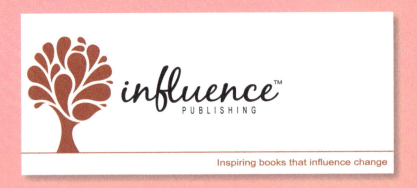

More information on our other titles and
how to submit your own proposal can be found at
www.InfluencePublishing.com

CPSIA information can be obtained at www.ICGtesting.com
Printed in the USA
LVOW021908120213

319715LV00004B/4/P